T0321185

INTERVENTIONS IN THE
ACUTE PHASE
OF MYOCARDIAL
INFARCTION

DEVELOPMENTS IN CARDIOVASCULAR MEDICINE

Lancee, C.T., ed.: Echocardiology, 1979. ISBN 90-247-2209-8.
Baan, J., Arntzenius, A.C., Yellin, E.L., eds.: Cardiac dynamics. 1980. ISBN 90-247-2212-8.
Thalen, H.J.T., Meere, C.C., eds.: Funadmentals of cardiac pacing. 1970. ISBN 90-247-2245-4.
Kulbertus, H.E., Wellens, H.J.J., eds.: Sudden death. 1980. ISBN 90-247-2290-X.
Dreifus, L.S., Brest, A.N., eds.: Clinical applications of cardiovascular drugs. 1980. ISBN 90-247-2295-0.
Spencer, M.P., Reid, J.M., eds.: Cerebrovascular evaluation with Doppler ultrasound. 1981. ISBN 90-247-90-247-2348-1.
Zipes, D.P., Bailey, J.C., Elharrar, V., eds.: The slow inward current and cardiac arrhythmias. 1980. ISBN 90-247-2380-9.
Kesteloot, H., Joossens, J.V., eds.: Epidemiology of arterial blood pressure. 1980. ISBN 90-247-2386-8.
Wackers, F.J.T., ed.: Thallium — 201 and technetium-99m-pyrophosphate myocardial imaging in the coronary care unit. 1980. ISBN 90-247-2396-5.
Maseri, A., Marchesi, C., Chierchia, S., Trivella, M.G., eds.: Coronary care units. 1981. ISBN 90-247-2456-2.
Morganroth, J., Moore, E.N., Dreifus, L.S., Michelson, E.L., eds.: The evaluation of new antiarrhythmic drugs. 1981. ISBN 90-247-2474-0.
Alboni, P.: Intraventricular conduction disturbances. 1981. ISBN 90-247-2483-X.
Rijsterborgh, H., ed.: Echocardiology. 1981. ISBN 90-247-2491-0.
Wagner, G.S., ed.: Myocardial infarction. Measurement and intervention. 1982. ISBN 90-247-2513-5.
Meltzer, R.S., Roelandt, J., eds.: Contrast echocardiography. 1982. ISBN 90-247-2531-3.
Amery, A., Fagard, R., Lijnen, R., Staessen, J., eds.: Hypertensive cardiovascular disease; pathophysiology and treatment. 1982. ISBN 90-247-2534-8.
Bouman, L.N., Jongsma, H.J., eds.: Cardiac rate and rhythm. 1982. ISBN 90-247-2626-3.
Morganroth, J., Moore, E.M., eds.: The evaluation of beta blockers and calcium antagonist drugs. 1982. ISBN 90-247-2642-5.
Rosenbaum, M.B., ed.: Frontiers of cardiac electrophysiology. 1982. ISBN 90-247-2663-8.
Roelandt, J., Hugenholtz, P.G., eds.: Long-term ambulatory electrocardiography. 1982. ISBN 90-247-2664-8.
Adgey, A.A.J., ed.: Acute phase of ischemic heart disease and myocardial infarction. 1982. ISBN 90-247-2675-1.
Hanrath, P., Bleifeld, W., Souguet, eds.: Cardiovascular diagnosis by ultrasound, ansesophageal, computerized, contrast, Doppler echocardiography. 1982. ISBN 90-247-2692-1.
Roelandt, J., ed.: The practice of M-mode and two-dimensional echocardiography. 1982. ISBN 90-247-2745-6.
Meyer, J., Schweizer, P., Erbel, R., eds.: Advances in non-invasive cardiology. ISBN 0-89838-576-8.
Perry, H.M., ed.: Life-long management of hypertension. ISBN 0-89838-572-2.
Jaffe, E.A., ed.: Biology of endothelial cells. ISBN 0-89838-587-3.
Surawicz, B., Reddy, C.P., Prystowsky, E.N., eds.: Tachycardiac. ISBN 0-89838-588-1.
Simoons, M.L., Reiber, J.H.C., eds.: Nuclear imaging in clinical cardiology. ISBN 0-89838-599-7.
Sperelakis, N., ed.: Physiology and pathophysiology of the heart. ISBN 0-89838-615-2.
Messerli, F.H., ed.: Kidney in essential hypertension. ISBN 0-89838-616-0.
Sambhi, M.P., ed.: Fundamental fault in hypertension. ISBN 0-89838-638-1.
Marchesi, C., ed.: Ambulatory monitoring: Cardiovascular system and allied applications. ISBN 0-89838-642-X.
Kupper, W., Macalpin, R.N., Bleifeld, W., eds.: Coronary tone in ischemic heart disease. ISBN 0-89838-646-2.
Sperelakis, N., Caulfield, J.B., eds.: Calcium antagonists: Mechanisms of action on cardiac muscle and vascular smooth muscle. ISBN 0-89838-655-1.
Godfraind, T., Herman, A.S., Wellens, D., eds.: Entry blockers in cardiovascular and cerebral dysfunctions. ISBN 0-89838-658-6.

INTERVENTIONS IN THE ACUTE PHASE OF MYOCARDIAL INFARCTION

Edited by

Joel Morganroth
E. Neil Moore

Martinus Nijhoff Publishing
A member of the Kluwer Academic Publishers Group
Boston/The Hague/Dordrecht/Lancaster

Distributors for North America:
Kluwer Academic Publishers
190 Old Derby Street
Hingham, MA 02043

Distributors Outside North America:
Kluwer Academic Publishers Group
Distribution Centre
P.O. Box 322
3300 AH Dordrecht
The Netherlands

Library of Congress Cataloging in Publication Data

Symposium on New Drugs and Devices (1983 : Philadelphia, Pa.)
   Interventions in the acute phase of myocardial infarction.

   (Developments in cardiovascular medicine)
   Includes bibliographical references.
   1. Heart—Infarction—Chemotherapy—Congresses. 2. Heart—Infarction—Treatment—
Congresses. I. Morganroth, Joel. II. Moore, E. Neil. III. Title. IV. Series. [DNLM:
1. Myocardial Infarction—drug therapy—congresses. 2. Myocardial Infarction—therapy—
congresses. W1 DE997VME / WG 300 S98925i 1983]
RC685.I6S88   1983   616.1'237   84-7972
ISBN 0-89838-659-4

Printed in the United States of America

CONTENTS

v

Devices to Limit Infarct Size

PREFACE

In the 1980's a primary focus for intense cardiovascular research is in the treatment of patients with acute myocardial infarction. Although the prevalence of this syndrome has been decreasing in the United States, still over 1.5 million patients develop myocardial infarction per year. There is about a 20% chance of a North American male developing myocardial infarction before the age of 65. The in-hospital mortality still remains at approximately 10%–15% and advances in pharmacologic and device therapy have allowed for the intensification of research in the treatment of patients with acute myocardial infarction.

The following manuscripts represent the collective efforts of academic investigators in the United States and abroad as well as members of the pharmaceutical industry, and the Food and Drug Administration to address the issues involved in interventions in the acute phase of myocardial infarction. State-of-the-art papers addressing important topics are followed by discussion sections which have allowed participants to express their own viewpoints leading to a consensus opinion. The first part of this Symposium addresses the models of experimental myocardial infarction followed by the important issue of how one defines myocardial infarction size. The latter is extremely important to be certain that endpoints of therapeutic or device interventions are objective and reproducible. A detailed description of the pharmacological interventions to reduce myocardial infarction size as well as newer devices to effect mechanical and electrical disorders provide an up-to-date summary of current opinion.

While we do not anticipate that this Symposium could evolve unanimous consensus opinions on many of the important issues raised, it is clear that important research concerns have been identified and suggestions for their solution have emerged.

We hope that this book will be helpful to those individuals who study the acute phase of myocardial infarction and hope it has provided guidelines, study design, and interpretation.

Joel Morganroth, M.D.
E. Neil Moore, D.V.M., Ph.D.

Philadelphia, Pennsylvania, U.S.A.

SYMPOSIUM ON NEW DRUGS AND DEVICES
October 6 and 7, 1983

FACULTY

Ronald W.F. Campbell, M.D.
Senior Lecturer and Consultant
Cardiologist
Freeman Hospital, England

Jay N. Cohn, M.D.
Professor of Medicine
University of Minnesota

Philip Dern, M.D.
Cardio-Renal Division
Food and Drug Administration

Stewart J. Ehrreich, Ph.D.
Deputy Director, Division of
Cardio-Renal Drug Products
Food and Drug Administration

Herman Gold, M.D.
Associate Professor of Medicine
Harvard Medical School

Sidney Goldstein, M.D.
Professor of Medicine
University of Michigan

Donald C. Harrison, M.D.
William G. Irwin Professor of Cardiology
Stanford University School of Medicine

Leonard N. Horowitz, M.D.
Associate Professor of Medicine
Hahnemann University

Jacob Kolff, M.D.
Professor of Surgery
Temple University School of Medicine

Raymond J. Lipicky, M.D.
Acting Director, Division of Cardio-
Renal Drug Products
Food and Drug Administration

Robert E. Keenan, M.D.
Vice-President, Medical Research
A.H. Robins Company, Inc.

Andrew Kemper, M.D.
Instructor in Medicine
Howard Medical School

Richard S. Kent, M.D.
Senior Clinical Research Scientist
Burroughs Wellcome Co.

Harris Koffer, Pharm.D.
Assistant Director
Philadelphia Association for
Clinical Trials

Jacob Kolff, M.D.
Professor of Surgery
Temple University Hospital

Ezra Lamdin, M.D.
Stuart Pharmaceuticals

David P. Lauler, M.D.
Chairman, Department of Medicine
Lawrence & Memorial Hospitals

Ralph Lazzara, M.D.
Professor of Medicine
University of Oklahoma Health
Sciences Center

xi

Robert J. Lee, Ph.D.
Vice President, Research & Development
American Critical Care

Jan Lessem, M.D.
Bristol-Myers Company

Raymond J. Lipicky, M.D.
Acting Director, Division of Cardio-Renal Drug Products
Food and Drug Administration

Henry S. Loeb, M.D.
Program Director in Cardiology
Veterans Administration Hospital

Margaret A. Longshore
Clinical Research Monitor
Ayerst Laboratories

Robert J. Loring, M.S.
Director of Research & Development
United Medical Corporation

E. Neil Moore, D.V.M., Ph.D.
Professor of Physiology in Medicine
University of Pennsylvania

Joel Morganroth, M.D.
Professor of Medicine and
Pharmacology
Hahnemann University

Glenn A. Rahmoeller
Director, Division of Cardiovascular
Devices
Food and Drug Administration

Keith A. Reimer, M.D., Ph.D.
Associate Professor of Medicine
Duke University Medical School

K. Peter Rentrop, M.D.
Associate Professor of Medicine
Mt. Sinai Medical Center

Peter Sleight, M.D.
Field-Marshall Alexander Professor of
Cardiovascular Medicine
University of Oxford, England

Burton E. Sobel, M.D.
Professor of Medicine
Washington University School
of Medicine

Robert Temple, M.D.
Acting Director, New Drug Evaluation
Food and Drug Administration

Zoltan Turi, M.D.
Assistant Professor of Medicine
Harvard Medical School

James Willerson, M.D.
Professor of Medicine
University of Texas Health Science
Center

Raymond L. Woosley, M.D., Ph.D.
Associate Professor of Medicine
and Pharmacology
Vanderbilt University Medical Center

INTERVENTIONS IN THE
ACUTE PHASE
OF MYOCARDIAL
INFARCTION

1

EXPERIMENTAL MODELS AND ENDPOINTS FOR EVALUATING INTERVENTIONS IN THE ACUTE PHASE OF MYOCARDIAL INFARCTION —AN ANATOMIC APPROACH

KEITH A. REIMER and ROBERT B. JENNINGS

1. INTRODUCTION

During the past decade and a half, investigators in many laboratories have been interested in assessing the effects of a variety of different interventions on acutely ischemic myocardium. It seems likely that the widespread interest in this problem has led to the development of more experimental models to study myocardial ischemia than there are laboratories conducting the studies. Table 1 lists a few of the potentially important variables among the various models which have been employed:

Table 1. MAJOR VARIABLES IN ANIMAL MODELS FOR TESTING INTERVENTIONS THAT MIGHT PROTECT ISCHEMIC MYOCARDIUM

SPECIES
ANESTHETIZED/AWAKE
INTACT ANIMAL/ISOLATED HEART/TISSUE CULTURE
ISCHEMIA/HYPOXIA
GLOBAL/REGIONAL ISCHEMIA
DURATION/SEVERITY OF INSULT
PERMANENT OCCLUSION/REPERFUSION
ONSET/DURATION/DOSE OF DRUG

For every model used, there must be one or more primary endpoints which are used to assess the effect of an intervention. The number of probable endpoints are perhaps even larger than the number of animal models employed (Table 2).

Each animal model and endpoint has certain advantages and limitations. It will not be possible to discuss the pros and cons of these different models or endpoints in this brief chapter. However, it is important to recognize the advantages and limitations of each so that, when a question is posed for study, the most appropriate model and endpoints will be chosen to answer the question.

Table 2. PRIMARY ENDPOINTS USED TO IDENTIFY POTENTIALLY BENEFICIAL EFFECTS OF INTERVENTION

INFARCT SIZE

—HISTOLOGIC

— GROSS/HISTOCHEMICAL

INDIRECT INDICES OF INFARCT SIZE IN VIVO
(ST SEGMENT/QRS MAPPING, ENZYME RELEASE CURVES, IMAGING TECHNIQUES, ETC).)

COLLATERAL BLOOD FLOW

MYOCARDIAL CONTRACTILE FUNCTION

ULTRASTRUCTURAL CHANGES

FUNCTION OF SUBCELLULAR ORGANELLES (IN INTACT OR FRACTIONATED CELLS)
(MITOCHONDRIA, SARCOPLASMIC RETICULUM, SARCOLEMMA, LYSOSOMES, ETC.)

BIOCHEMICAL CHANGES
(HIGH ENERGY PHOSPHATES, pH, ION GRADIENTS, CATABOLITES, ETC.)

General considerations that aid in the selection of a particular model are listed in Table 3. Some models may be far removed from clinical reality but because of simplicity and/or ease of interpretation may nevertheless be useful for identifying potentially useful therapies from the large number of possible interventions available for study. On the other hand, more complicated and costly models designed to reproduce certain clinical conditions may be useful for preclinical study of the relatively few interventions that prove to be effective in simpler screening studies.

Table 3. CRITERIA FOR SELECTING ANIMAL MODELS AND ENDPOINTS
EXPERIMENTAL MODEL -
    SIMPLE SCREENING MODELS VS.
    COMPLEX MODELS TO REPRODUCE CLINICAL CONDITIONS
PRIMARY ENDPOINT(S) -
    QUESTION UNDER TEST
    ACCURACY VS. SIMPLICITY
SECONDARY VARIABLES -
    CONTROL FOR VARIATION IN PRIMARY ENDPOINTS

The choice of primary endpoints should be based on the question under test. For example, if the question is "Will drug 'X' preserve or improve myocardial function following myocardial infarction?", a measure of myocardial function is needed. Measurement of infarct size will not provide an answer to the question except in the broad sense that dead muscle will never resume contractile activity. Conversely, if the specific question is "Will drug 'X' limit infarct size?", the endpoint should be infarct size and not indirect indices of infarct size such as ECG parameters, enzyme release curves or measures of myocardial function. In clinical studies, infarct size must be inferred from one or more indirect indices of infarct size because direct measurement is not possible. However, in experimental studies in which infarct size is the primary endpoint of interest, there seldom is any rationale for using indirect indices to estimate infarct size.

With any experimental model, there will be biologic variation in the primary endpoint. In order to tighten up an experimental model as much as possible, the major determinants of variation in the primary endpoint should be identified and these determinants should be measured as secondary endpoints to control for variation in the primary endpoints. For example, in the anesthetized dog, two very important determinants of infarct size are the size of the ischemic vascular bed and collateral blood flow (1-5).

2. EVOLUTION OF ACUTE MYOCARDIAL INFARCTS IN OPEN CHEST DOGS

We have developed several experimental models to test whether an intervention can limit infarct size, based on studies we did several years ago to evaluate the time course of the development of a myocardial infarct following occlusion of the circumflex artery in open chest dogs (3). In those studies, anesthetized dogs with left thoracotomies were used. Forty minutes, three hours, and six hours of temporary occlusion of the circumflex artery were compared with four days of permanent occlusion. The dogs with temporary ischemia were reperfused by removal of the occluding snare and all dogs were allowed to recover and were killed for study on the fourth day. The primary endpoint was infarct size, measured by histologic techniques. Secondary endpoints were the size of the occluded vascular bed, collateral flow in transmural thirds of the central ischemic region, and hemodynamic parameters such as heart rate and blood pressure.

Following proximal occlusion of a major coronary artery in the open chest dog, there virtually always is a transmural gradient of collateral blood flow (Figure 1), so that the subendocardial (inner) region is severely ischemic (flow < .15 ml/min/gm) while the subepicardial region is less ischemic and often exhibits moderate quantities of collateral flow, i.e. .15 to .30 ml/min/gm (6-9). However, the amount of collateral flow, particularly to the subepicardial region, varies markedly among dogs.

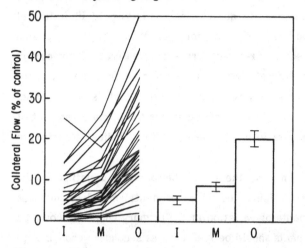

Figure 1. The transmural distribution of collateral flow found 20 minutes after circumflex occlusion in 31 dogs. Flow was measured with 9+1 μm microspheres before and after coronary occlusion. Collateral flow is expressed as a percentage of preocclusion flow to the same samples. The individual dogs are illustrated on the left and the group means + SEM are shown on the right. I, M, and O = inner, middle, and outer thirds of the transmural wall in the circumflex bed. Subendocardial flow was almost always severely depressed (<15%) and averaged 4.5% of control. Subepicardial flow was greater (averaged 20% of control) and much more variable than subendocardial flow. Reproduced from reference 3 with permission of the publisher.

The time of onset of irreversible cell injury correlates with the severity of ischemia (Figure 2). With reperfusion at 40 minutes, only the severely ischemic subendocardial region dies. Moreover, in the subendocardial region, lateral boundaries of the infarct are determined by the boundaries of the occluded vascular bed. The outer, more moderately ischemic subepicardial region is spared by reperfusion. Reperfusion after three hours of ischemia is associated with more extensive infarcts but some of the moderately ischemic subepicardial region still is salvaged at this time. In the absence of reperfusion, in the center of the ischemic bed, infarcts are nearly transmural. Thus, there is a transmural progression of irreversible injury — a spreading wavefront of cell death —with increasing duration of occlusion (3).

3.   ASSESSING POSSIBLE LIMITATION OF INFARCT SIZE IN OPEN CHEST DOGS

Given this biology of myocardial infarction in the open chest dog, we have used three different models to evaluate the effects of interventions (Table 4). These three models differ technically primarily in the duration of ischemia but

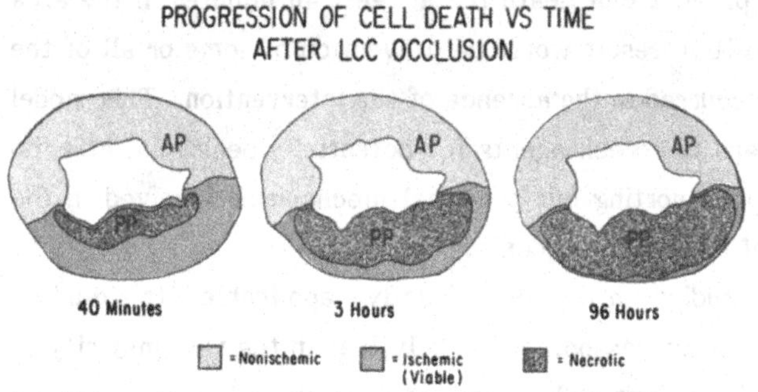

FIGURE 2. Progression of cell death vs. time after left circumflex coronary artery occlusion. Necrosis occurs first in the subendocardial myocardium. With longer occlusions, a wavefront of cell death moves from the subendocardial zone across the wall to involve progressively more of the transmural thickness of the ischemic zone. In contrast, the lateral margins in the subendocardial region of the infarct are established as early as 40 minutes after occlusion and are sharply defined by the anatomic boundaries of the ischemic bed. AP = anterior papillary muscle; PP = posterior papillary muscle. Reproduced from reference 3 with permission of the publisher.

Table 4. RATIONALE OF MODELS TO STUDY THE EFFECT OF INTERVENTIONS ON MYOCARDIAL ISCHEMIC CELL DEATH IN ANESTHETIZED DOGS.

MODEL: 40 MINUTE TEMPORARY CORONARY OCCLUSION (FOUR DAYS REPERFUSION).

PURPOSE: TO DETECT DELAY OF CELL DEATH IN THE SUBENDOCARDIAL ZONE OF SEVERE ISCHEMIA.

MODEL: 3 HOUR TEMPORARY CORONARY OCCLUSION (FOUR DAYS REPERFUSION)

PURPOSE: TO DETECT DELAY OF CELL DEATH IN THE MID/SUBEPICARDIAL ZONE OF MODERATE ISCHEMIA.

MODEL: PERMANENT (FOUR DAYS) CORONARY LIGATION

PURPOSE: TO DETECT ABSOLUTE LIMITATION OF INFARCT SIZE (PREVENTION OF CELL DEATH) IN THE MID/SUBEPICARDIAL ZONE OF MODERATE ISCHEMIA

the rationale differs importantly among the models. If we want to know whether an intervention will delay the onset of lethal cell injury in severely ischemic myocardium, we use a 40 minute period of ischemia followed by reperfusion. In this setting the moderately ischemic subepicardial region will survive because of reperfusion. Thus with this model, the question under test is whether an intervention can delay or prevent cell death for at least 40 minutes in the area of severe ischemia. A positive result would be prevention of some or all of the necrosis that would have occurred in the absence of the intervention. This model provides the simplest means to screen agents for potentially beneficial effects. It also is especially useful in sorting out potential mechanisms involved in the subcellular pathogenesis of ischemic cell death.

Results of such studies are not directly applicable to clinical circumstances, for the following reason. It is likely that in the vast majority of patients, severely ischemic regions will be beyond salvage by the time therapy can be started. Thus, the goal clinically must be to salvage some of the moderately ischemic myocardium in the subepicardial region and thereby to convert a potentially transmural infarct into a more subendocardial infarct. It is logical to hypothesize that an intervention which delays cell death in severely ischemic regions also should delay cell death in moderately ischemic regions, but this hypothesis remains unproven.

To evaluate the effect of an intervention on moderately ischemic myocardium, we use a three hour period of ischemia followed by reperfusion. By three hours, much, but not quite all of the myocardium destined to become necrotic (infarcted) has already been irreversibly injured. Thus, an intervention that delays cell death in the moderately ischemic subepicardial region should result in limitation of the transmural extent of infarct in this model.

This model is most directly applicable clinically to situations in which early reperfusion is established, e.g., by streptokinase, transluminal angioplasty, or emergency bypass surgery. Maneuvers to establish reperfusion could be preceded by immediate drug intervention when the patient first was evaluated in the hospital emergency room. In addition, patients known to have significant coronary artery disease and to be at risk of myocardial infarction could be chronically treated with an agent known to delay myocardial ischemic injury.

In order to determine whether an intervention has a sustained protective effect on ischemic myocardium, a permanent occlusion model is required. With a permanent occlusion model, absolute limitation of infarct size can be detected. However, by comparison with the three hour model, the permanent occlusion model is a more difficult and more costly experimental design. In the three hour model, ischemic injury occurs during a finite time period in which therapy can be continuously administered, hemodynamics closely monitored, and the severity of ischemia measured. With permanent occlusions, long term therapy and hemodynamic monitoring may be required. For this reason, it is much more efficient to establish the effectiveness of therapy in a reperfusion model before testing an intervention in a permanent model of infarction. An intervention that delays cell death in the three hour reperfusion model may or may not effect an absolute limitation in infarct size. Conversely, we believe that any intervention which cannot delay injury for at least three hours is not worth evaluating in a long term occlusion study.

In each of these models, our primary endpoint is infarct size, which we measure from histologic sections of the heart (Table 5) (3). Other investigators measure infarct size based on nitro-blue tetrazolium or triphenyl-tetrazolium chloride staining techniques which are less costly and less time consuming but also in our experience, less reliable than histologic techniques.

Table 5. ENDPOINTS TO EVALUATE THE EFFECT OF INTERVENTIONS ON MYOCARDIAL ISCHEMIC CELL DEATH IN ANESTHETIZED DOGS

PRIMARY END POINT: INFARCT SIZE

SECONDARY VARIABLES WHICH INFLUENCE INFARCT SIZE:

    1.   ANATOMIC SIZE OF THE OCCLUDED VASCULAR BED AT RISK

    2.   INTRINSIC COLLATERAL FLOW AVAILABLE TO THE ISCHEMIC REGION.

    3.   HEMODYNAMIC DETERMINANTS OF METABOLIC DEMAND, E.G., HEART RATE AND BLOOD PRESSURE.

The major determinants of infarct size in the absence of therapy are the size of the ischemic region and the amount of collateral blood flow within this ischemic region. Hemodynamic parameters such as heart rate and blood pressure also may influence infarct size and these factors all are measured to control for variation in the primary endpoint, i.e., infarct size (3,14). The size of the occluded vascular bed can be measured from gross photographs following simultaneous post-mortem perfusion of the coronary arteries with colored dyes (3) or from post mortem x-rays taken after coronary injection with barium sulphate (2,15). Collateral blood flow is measured with microspheres (3).

In untreated dogs, the transmural extent of an infarct is inversely related to collateral blood flow (3). Figure 3 is a schematic illustration of how the relationship between infarct size and collateral blood flow can be used to evaluate the effect of therapy. With an intervention that limits infarct size without altering collateral blood flow, infarcts should be smaller for any level of collateral flow and the regression line of infarct size vs. flow would be shifted downward (left panel). On the other hand, a therapy that improved collateral blood flow could limit infarct size by moving points down the regression line (right panel). Thus, incorporation of collateral flow measurements should 1) permit detection of a positive effect with greater precision and 2) provide information about the mechanism of treatment effect.

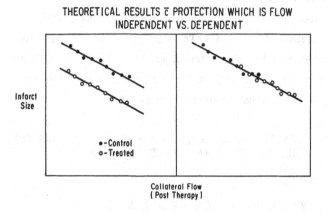

THEORETICAL RESULTS c̄ PROTECTION WHICH IS FLOW
INDEPENDENT VS. DEPENDENT

Infarct Size

•–Control
o–Treated

Collateral Flow
(Post Therapy)

FIGURE 3. Schematic illustration of the effect of interventions which limit infarct size on the regression of infarct size vs. collateral blood flow. See text for explanation.

The advantage of this analysis is best illustrated in our reperfusion studies in which infarct size was measured four days after 40 minutes, three hours, or six hours of temporary occlusion and compared with infarct size four days after permanent ligation of the circumflex artery. Permanent occlusion resulted in infarcts averaging about 40% of the left ventricle and 80% of the occluded vascular bed (Figure 4). Reperfusion after 40 minutes clearly limited infarct size to about 13% of the left ventricle and 28% of the myocardium at risk. Reperfusion at three hours or 6 hours both appeared to limit infarct size slightly.

A more precise analysis of the effect of reperfusion at these times was achieved by plotting the transmural extent of infarction against collateral flow to the subepicardial zone of the ischemic region (Figure 5). Infarcts reperfused at six hours were similar to permanent infarcts. However, the regression line was clearly shifted downward by reperfusion at three hours. Thus, at any level of collateral flow, reperfusion at three hours limited infarct size. Without the measurement of collateral blood flow, this protective effect was barely detectable and rather unconvincing. Conversely the slight but statistically significant limitation of infarct size with reperfusion at six hours shown on Figure 4 was, in fact, an artifact due to random selection into this group of several dogs with relatively high native collateral flow.

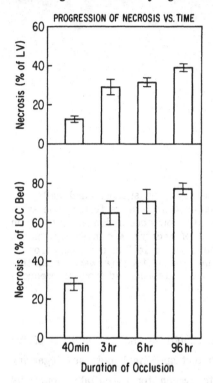

FIGURE 4. Infarct size (± SEM) with increasing duration of coronary occlusion. Means are expressed as a percent of the left ventricle (top) or percent of the circumflex bed identified by postmortem coronary perfusion techniques (bottom). Forty minutes to 6 hours of ischemia followed by 96 hours of reperfusion are compared with 96-hour-old infarcts that were not reperfused. Infarct size after reperfusion was significantly smaller (p< .05) at all times compared with permanent infarcts. However, the magnitude of the difference was small at 3 and 6 hours. Based on the data from table 2 in reference 3.

This example illustrates how important measurements of collateral blood flow are in this type of experiment. Because native collateral flow is so variable in dogs it would be easy with the relatively small groups of dogs commonly studied to select several dogs with unusually high or low flow. Because flow is a strong determinant of infarct size, such selection could result either in failure to detect a positive effect of intervention or in detection of an artifactually positive result.

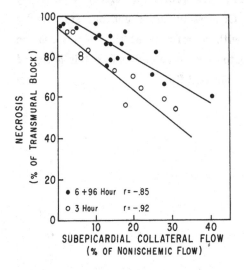

FIGURE 5   Relation between transmural necrosis and subepicardial collateral flow.   Permanent infarcts and infarcts reperfused at 6 hours formed the same line and were combined. Infarcts reperfused at 3 hours are indicated by the open circles. In both groups, the transmural extent of necrosis was inversely related to subepicardial flow measured at 20 minutes after left circumflex coronary occlusion. However, the 3 hour regression line was shifted downward, indicating that reperfusion at 3 hours limited infarct size. Reproduced from reference 3 with permission of the publisher.

4.   SUMMARY

The choice of an experimental model should depend on the goals of the study.   Simple models should be chosen to test specific hypotheses regarding mechanisms of ischemic cell injury and to screen for potentially beneficial interventions. More complex models should be used for preclinical testing. The primary endpoint(s) should depend on the specific question under test and secondary variables should be measured to control for variation in the primary endpoint(s). In dog models used to determine whether an intervention limits infarct size, an anatomic assessment of infarct size should be the primary endpoint.   Secondary variables should include the two major variable determinants of infarct size, i.e. a) the size of the occluded vascular bed and b) the amount of collateral blood flow within the subepicardial zone of this anatomic area at risk, as well as hemodynamic determinants of myocardial metabolic demand.

REFERENCES

1. Lowe JE, Reimer KA, Jennings RB: Experimental infarct size as a function of the amount of myocardium at risk. Am J Pathol (90):363-380, 1978.
2. Jugdutt BI, Hutchins GM, Bulkley BH, Becker LC: Myocardial infarction in the conscious dog: Three dimensional mapping of infarct, collateral flow, and region at risk. Circulation (60): 1141-1150, 1979.
3. Reimer KA, Jennings RB. The "Wavefront Phenomenon" of myocardial ischemic cell death. II. Transmural progression of necrosis within the framework of ischemic bed size (myocardium at risk) and collateral flow. Lab Invest (40):633-644, 1979.
4. Rivas F, Cobb FR, Bache RJ, Greenfield JC, Jr.: Relationship between blood flow to ischemic regions and extent of myocardial infarction. Serial measurement of blood flow to ischemic regions in dogs. Circ Res (38):439-447, 1976.
5. Schaper W: Experimental coronary artery occlusion. III. The determinants of collateral blood flow in acute coronary occlusion. Basic Res Cardiol (73):584-594, 1978.
6. Becker LC, Ferreira R, Thomas M: Mapping of left ventricular blood flow with radioactive microspheres in experimental coronary artery occlusion. Cardiovasc Res (7):391-400, 1973.
7. Bishop SP, White FC, Bloor CM: Regional myocardial blood flow during acute myocardial infarction in the conscious dog. Circ Res (38):429-438, 1976.
8. Kloner RA, Reimer KA, Jennings RB: Distribution of collateral flow in acute myocardial ischemic injury—effect of propranolol therapy. Cardiovasc Res (10):81-90, 1976.
9. Schaper W, Pasyk S: Influence of collateral flow on the ischemic tolerance of the heart following acute and subacute coronary occlusion. Circulation (53): I-57-I-62, 1976.
10. Jennings, RB and Reimer KA: Biology of experimental acute myocardial ischemia and infarction. In Hearse, DJ and DeLeiris J (eds.) Enzymes in Cardiology. Diagnosis and Research. John Wiley & Sons, New York, 1979, pp. 21-57.
11. Lie JT, Pairolero PC, Holley KE, Titus JL: Macroscopic enzyme-mapping verification of large, homogeneous, experimental myocardial infarcts of predictable size and location in dogs. J Thorac Cardiovasc Surg (69): 599-605, 1975.
12. Fishbein MC, Meerbaum S, Rit J, Lando U, Kanmatsuse K, Mercier JC, Corday E, Ganz W: Early phase acute myocardial infarct size quantification: validation of the triphenyl tetrazolium chloride technique. Am Heart J (101): 593-600, 1981.
13. Schaper W, Frenzel H, Hort W: Experimental coronary artery occlusion. I. Measurement of infarct size. Basic Res Cardiol (74): 46-53, 1979.
14. Schaper W: Residual perfusion of acutely ischemic heart muscle. In: Schaper, W. (ed) The Pathophysiology of Myocardial Perfusion. Elsevier/North-Holland Biomedical Press, 1979, pp. 345-378.
15. Lee JT, Ideker RE, Reimer KA: Myocardial infarct size and location in relation to the coronary vascular bed at risk in man. Circulation (64): 526-534, 1981.

2

MODELS TO STUDY EXPERIMENTAL INFARCTION - PHARMACOLOGIC

Stewart J. Ehrreich, Ph.D.
Food and Drug Administration

1. INTRODUCTION

A new drug generally cannot be found without an appropriate animal model to be used for the discovery and development phases. The only exceptions are compounds found to be active as a result of particular clinical experiences. Most of the time such experiences uncover new indications for an old drug. Recent examples of this are studies which tested the hypothesis that use of beta-blocking agents in patients who had a previous myocardial infarction might be beneficial in preventing death.

Could an animal model have predicted the same outcome?

Not likely, but the myocardial salvage properties of beta-blockers in an acute experiments has already been demonstrated. The long term predictive value however, of such models is not yet clear at the present time.

2. ANIMAL MODELS FOR MI. - WHAT ARE THE PURPOSES?

Animal models for MI have several uses. They can be used to test for activity in the following:

2.1.1. Cardiac arrhythmias

2.1.2. Angina

2.1.3. Cardiac ischemia (including effects on blood flow)

2.1.4. Prevention/reduction of cardiac cell loss (reduce infarct size)

2.1.5. Positive inotropy

For the purposes of this discussion, item (e) above (models of experimental heart failure) will not be addressed.

A large number of animal models are available to fulfill the needs for new drug discovery and evaluation. Their relevance to the clinical situation is always uncertain. The ability to "discover" a new agent in these models must be confirmed by testing in man before some credibility factor can be assigned to the model.

The ability of the model to detect already proved clinically useful agents ("standards") is required before trust can be placed in the procedure. Sometimes a new model which is not capable of such detection appears theoretically valuable and may be able to detect new mechanisms for treatment. Further development of such models has to be based on trust and a strong scientific base.

The MI models currently have their largest use in the screening and evaluation of antiarrhythmic agents. This is because the arrhythmias resulting from experimental coronary occlusion are largely the re-entry type and mimic the more serious and potentially life threatening arrhythmias which are observed clinically in MI patients.

Drug sponsors are also more likely to test drugs for antiarrhythmic properties, not only because the medical need and market potential are evident, but the clinical trials for antiarrhythmic agents are more clearly defined, are more manageable, with relatively small numbers of patients, and may quickly predict efficacy and safety. Their cost is miniscule by comparison to long range infarction trials.

Likewise, therapeutic trials in patients who have various types and severity of arrhythmias continue to be published and a wide variety of "new standard" agents can be tested in the models as a method to compare experimental agents for relative potential clinical utility and to help validate the model for its predictive ability in this situation.

Partly because of the unknown carry-over of beneficial effects in animal models of myocardial infarction to man, many of these models have not found a solid place in the screening procedures used in the pharmaceutical industry. Also, many of these models are difficult to prepare, time consuming and very costly. Quite a few use larger animals such as dogs and pigs and several animal preparations need to be successfully used in order to test a single compound. While therapeutic efficacy is difficult and of questionable value, prophylactic trials in animal models are even more unreliable and the drug industry generally does not consider using such models at present. Furthermore, potential prophylactic trials in man is a nightmare to be avoided. Papers have been published recently (Marshall et al, 1980) indicating that lidocaine infusions prior to coronary ligation in greyhounds reduced the incidence of ventricular PVS's but not fibrillation. This may indicate that lidocaine is only effective when given therapeutically, not a totally unexpected finding.

Publications over the last 10 to 15 years have also caused the investigator who uses animal models to be more insecure since data have shown that some compounds "active" in animal models such as coronary vasodilators like persantine and salvage agents such as steroids may be not only inactive clinically but potentially dangerous. A long term trial to test the ability of steroids in myocardial infarction is presently underway.

In our own FDA laboratories our group headed by Tibor Balazs, Gordon Johnson and myself have studied a rat model of catecholamine-induced cardiac necrosis which behaves in a fashion not dissimilar to man and which seems sensitive to various classes of compounds. Some discussion about this model will be made later on in this presentation.

As mentioned briefly before, the limiting factor for model development in industry has been the understandable reluctance of management to pursue a particular investigational compound on the strength of results in a single model or even two or more models when:

2.2.1. Few animals/tissues were actually used for verification of activity.

2.2.2. Only in vitro tests form the basis for interest in the compound.

2.2.3. Solubility of the test substance is an important factor, especially in in vitro testing, limiting tests to water soluble compounds only.

2.2.4. Secondary or tertiary validating models may not exist, or may be even less reliable.

2.2.5. There is a fear that a "thin" pharmacologic profile (not the toxicity studies) will not "pass" FDA muster.

2.2.6. The cost and time required of clinical trials is too great to warrant the financial commitment, as mentioned above.

Based on the present literature, I know of no compound in clinical trials which reached that stage of development as a result solely of MI prevention/reduction in an experimental animal model. All current investigational agents are either antiarrhythmic or beta-blocking or have calcium-antagonist properties and have been tested in more accepted and reliable models for those effects. Some of these agents possessing these characteristics have been tested in MI models, but only to determine if they have other important properties.

3. TYPES OF ANIMAL MODELS FOR MI

While there are many, only a few are discussed here. Current models, of which the first four are the most widely used at present, are listed below:

3.1. Arteriosclerotic: food or chemical induced (Guinea Pig, primate, rabbit, etc).

3.2. Catecholamine-induced: Isoproterenol or other sympathomimetic agent which causes myocardial cell necrosis (rat).

3.3. Acute ligation or stenosis: (Anesthetized); primates, pig, dog, cat.

3.4. Acute/chronic ligation or stenosis: Conscious animal (survival); pig, dog, cat, rabbit, rat.

3.5. Isolated Tissues: various animals.

3.6. Organ culture: fetal mouse, chick embryo.

3.7. Cell culture: chick embryo; individual myocardial fibers.

4. CORONARY OCCLUSION MODELS

Various models of experimental coronary occlusion in animals as the baboon have shown to be insensitive to such drugs as nifedipine (Geary, et al, 1982). Diltiazem (Patterson, et al, 1982) has shown to be ineffective in various dog models as well. Verapamil, the benchmark calcium antagonist has been shown to be effective in preventing re-entrant activity in tissues from hearts of infarcted dogs, (Dersham, et al, 1981) probably by inhibition of slow responses in damaged myocardium. Likewise the drug has shown to reduce infarct size in dogs. (DeBoer, et al, 1980).

These models have the perplexing feature of variability of size and placement of the infarct dependent upon the size of the vessel occluded and degree of coronary collateralization. It is well known that the dog has a high degree of collateral development while the baboon and pig (or minipig) do not. Thus the latter models may be more similar to man and may be better predictors for human use and this has been discussed by many investigtors over the last two decades.

4.1 Experimental Thrombosis:

Coronary occlusion studies in which occlusion is produced by electrical stimulation of blood vessal walls causing an occlusive thrombosis have shown that non-steroidal antiinflammatory agents may prevent such thrombosis (Hook, et al, 1983). The closest attempt at an answer to potential clinical efficacy for the drugs has been the aspirin and anturane trials which have not been able to demonstrate clear clinical efficacy.

Molsidimine, an experimental agent has shown positive results in similar coronary artery thrombosis experiments (Fiedler, 1981) but clinical data supporting this finding is not yet published.

4.2 Catecholamine-induced cardiac necrosis

Several recent communications by our group (Johnson, et al, 1980; Ehrreich, et al, 1981; Johnson, et al, 1983; Ehrreich, et al, 1983; Balazs, et al, 1983; Kojima, et al, 1983) have shown that isoproterenol may be used to produce experimental cardiac necrosis which has interesting characteristics.

Early work by many investigators has already demonstrated the sensitivity of the myocardium to lesion producing actions of catecholamines. Many papers from the laboratories of Rona, Lehr and Balazs (among others) over the last two decades have brought interest in this model. Our interest was peaked when we found that vasodilator drugs which cause endogenous release of catecholamines (such as minoxidil and hydralazine) also cause experimental cardiac lesions. (Balazs, et al, 1981, 1982)

Our recent studies into the investigation of such a a pharmacologic model of MI has shown that small doses of isoproterenol (less than 0.5 mg/kg) produces ventricular fibrillation in rats weighing about 500 grams. Surviving animals have cardiac lesions whose severity is roughly proportional to dose of catecholamine administered.

Such animals are offered marked protection by moderate doses of beta-blocking agents but not calcium antagonists. Small infarction-producing doses of isoproterenol (approximately 0.05 mg/kg S.C.) protect animals from further larger doses of drug. A calorically restricted diet which reduces body weight by 10% is also effective and the protective effects last for a significant time period even after refeeding.

We are currently investigating the mechanisms of the small dose isoproterenol protection as well as diet on the survivability of these animals. Smaller (lighter but not necessarily younger) rats of about 200-300 grams have over a 1,000-fold greater tolerance to isoproterenol, and die not of ventricular fibrillation but respiratory arrest. Such animals also have cardiac lesions whose severity seems to be less than the heavier animals.

We are investigating whether the stress of diet, its nutritional characteristics or small doses of agonist can produce metabolic conditions in which large insults to the myocardium can be rebuffed by these animals. Since the protective effects occur quickly and heart weights are not affected, revascularization and altered hemodynamics may not be mechanisms for the resistance phenomenon. Further, our experiments indicate that the protective effect of the various interventions discussed above may have long lasting properties indicating a potential biochemical or metabolic alteration at the cellular level.

The model seems also be be sensitive to certain antifibrillatory agents and may behave similarly to man with regard to post myocardial infarction arrhythmias. Biochemical investigations are underway under the direction of a Visiting Professor, Dr. Sigmund Gudbjarnason who is an expert in cardiac lipids and myocardial metabolism.

While no one model of myocardial cell damage may be predictive of the clinical situation in man, such experiments take us closer not only to new drugs but to a better understanding of the cardiac ischemia-arrhythmia phenomena.

1. Marshall, R. J. and Parratt, J. R. Prophylactic lignocaine and early post-coronary artery occlusion dysrhythmias in anesthetized greyhounds. Br. J. Pharmacol. 71, 597, 1980.
2. Geary, G. G., Smith, G. T., Suehiro, G. T. and McNamara, J. J. Failure of nifedipine therapy to reduce myocardial infarct size in the baboon. Amer. J. Cardiol. 49, 331, 1982.
3. Patterson, E., Eller, B. T. and Lucchesi, B. R. Effects of diltiazem upon experimental ventricular dysrhythmias. J. Pharmacol. Exp. Ther. 225, 224, 1983.
4. Dersham, G. H. and Han, J. Actions of verapamil on purkinje fibers from normal and infarcted heart tissues. J. Pharmacol. Exp. Ther. 216, 261, 1981.
5. DeBoer, L. W., Strauss, H. W., Kloner, R. A., Rude, R. E., Davis, R. F., Maroko, P. R. and Braunwald, E. Autoradiographic method for measuring the ischemic myocardium at risk: Effects of verapamil on infarct size after experimental coronary occlusion. Proc. Nat. Acad. Sci. 77(10), 6119, 1980.
6. Hook, B. G., Romson, J. L., Jolly, S. R., Bailie, M. B. and Luchessi, B. R. Effect of Zomepirac on experimental coronary artery thrombosis and ischemic myocardial injury in the conscious dog. J. Cardiovasc. Pharmacol. 5, 302, 1983.
7. Fiedler, V. B. Effects of molsidomine on coronary artery thrombosis and myocardial ischemia in acute canine experiments. Euro. Jour. Pharmacol. 73, 85, 1981.
8. Johnson, G., Balazs, T., Ehrreich, S. J., Kenimer, J. G. and Bloom, S. On the resistance to isoproterenol induced cardiomyopathy in rats. Fed. Proc. 39:308, 1980.
9. Ehrreich, S. J., Johnson, G. L., Bloom, S. and Balazs, T. Isoproterenol toxicity in rats as a function of changes in body weight. The Pharmacologist 23:115, 1981.
10. Johnson, G., Ehrreich, S., El-Hage, A. and Balazs, T. Effect of antiarrhythmic agents on isoproterenol-induced ventricular fibrillation in heavy rats: A possible model of Sudden Death. Abstract; II World Conference on Clinical Pharmacology and Therapeutics, January 1983.
11. Ehrreich, S., Johnson, G., Kojima, M., Sperelakis, N., Whitehurst, V. and Balazs, T. Pharmacologic Biochemical and Electrophysiologic Responses of the Myocardium of Rats Subjects to Toxic Doses of Isoproterenol. Toxicology Letters, Vol. 18, Suppl. 1, 18, 1983.
12. Balazs, T., Johnson, G., Joseph, X., Ehrreich, S., and Bloom, S. Sensitivity and resistance of the myocardium to the toxicity of isoproterenol in rats. In: Myocardial Injury John J. Spitzer, Ed. Plenum Publishing Corp., 1983.
13. Kojima M., Sperelakis, N., Johnson, G., Ehrreich, S. and Balazs, T. Age-Dependent Changes in Electrophysiologic Characteristics of Fast and Slow Action Potentials in Rat Papillary Muscle. Accepted for publication: Canadian J. of Physiol., 1983.

14. Balazs, T., Ferrans, V. J., El-Hage, A., Ehrreich, S. J., Johnson, G. L., Herman, E. H., Atkinson, J. C. and West, W. L. Study on the mechanism of hydralazine-induced myocardial necrosis in the rat. Toxicol. Appl. Pharmacol. 59:524, 1981.

15. Balazs, T. and Bloom, S. Cardiotoxicity of Adrenergic Bronchodilator and Vasodilating Antihypertensive Drugs. In: Cardiovascular Toxicology, E. W. VanStee, Ed., Raven Press, N.Y. 1982, p. 199.

3

PHARMACOKINETICS OF ANTI-ARRHYTHMIC AGENTS IN ACUTE
MYOCARDIAL INFARCTION

RAYMOND L. WOOSLEY, M.D., Ph.D., IRENE CERSKUS, Ph.D., and
DAN M. RODEN, M.D.

Departments of Medicine and Pharmacology
Vanderbilt University School of Medicine, Nashville, Tennessee

SUMMARY

It is becoming increasingly apparent that the pharmacokinetics of many anti-arrhythmic agents are altered when administered to patients with acute myocardial infarction. Absorption following oral dosing may be delayed or incomplete. Volume of distribution, renal and hepatic clearance may be decreased due to diminished cardiac output and poor organ perfusion. Elimination half-life may be prolonged. Plasma protein binding may be dramatically increased due to elevated levels of alpha-1-acid glycoprotein, with attendant changes in drug total plasma concentration and levels of free drug. Delivery of drug to the ischemic myocardium may be slowed, with poorly-perfused regions functioning as "peripheral compartments". In some cases, however, pharmacokinetics appear relatively undisturbed after acute myocardial infarction.

Drugs likely to be used in patients with myocardial infarction should be evaluated in this setting, as extrapolation of pharmaco-kinetic data obtained in other subjects may be inappropriate.

Acute myocardial infarction (MI) presents a special challenge to the physician. The patient is in an unstable condition, often presenting with potentially life-threatening arrhythmias requiring treatment, or perhaps prophylaxis against such arrhythmias. Mortality is highest in the initial hours following infarction, although the patient remains highly vulnerable for some time thereafter (1). Most deaths are a result of ventricular fibrillation which may, or may not, be preceded by "warning arrhythmias" (2). In any event, many patients with MI will, at some time soon following their initial symptoms, receive anti-arrhythmic therapy. If such therapy is to be effective, with minimal adverse effects, an understanding of the drugs' pharmacokinetics can be invaluable in determining appropriate dosage and frequency of administration.

Pharmacokinetic profiles are usually established early in a new drug's development, and such studies are most often performed in healthy volunteers. It is becoming increasingly apparent, however, that pharmacokinetic variables may be altered in acute MI. Furthermore, such alterations may result in unique handling of the drug, with pharmacokinetic variables quite distinct from those obtained in patients with more stable illness. Before discussing the pharmacokinetics of anti-arrhythmic drugs in acute MI, a brief review of pharmacokinetic principles may be helpful.

Pharmacokinetics describes the time course of the absorption, distribution and elimination of a drug in the body while pharmacodynamics explores the relationship between drug dose and response. Together these data enable dosing guidelines to be established and determine the therapeutic range for a drug. Variables of interest include the volume of distribution, absorption and elimination half-life, bioavailability and clearance.

The volume of distribution is a concept which aids in determining the disposition of a drug in the body, and is estimated by dividing the dose administered by the plasma concentration extrapolated to time zero. The "volume" does not necessarily correspond to any physiologic space. For instance, a drug which is extensively tissue bound will have only a small fraction of the dose in the plasma, and therefore the total volume of distribution will be very large; far in excess of total body water.

The systemic bioavailability of a drug is that portion of the dose administered which enters the systemic circulation. Drugs may have low bioavailability due to poor absorption, or they may be subject to metabolism in the liver or, less commonly, the gut wall, before entering the general circulation. Bioavailability is usually determined by comparing the area under the plasma concentration–time curve (AUC) after oral administration to that after intravenous administration (by definition, 100% bioavailable).

Absorption and elimination half-life describe the time-course of entry to and exit from the vascular compartment. Half-life, by definition, is the time taken for half of these processes to be complete. Approximately five elimination half-lives are required to achieve steady state conditions at which time the amount of drug entering the system is balanced by the amount eliminated. Elimination most often occurs via metabolism in the liver and/or renal excretion.

The clearance of a drug refers to its rate of removal from plasma. Changes in protein binding may or may not influence the clearance of a drug. Since, in the absence of an active transport system, bound drug is unable to cross cell membranes, changes in protein binding will affect the clearance of drugs which are eliminated by glomerular filtration or passive diffusion to hepatic sites of metabolism. On the other hand, drugs which are cleared by renal tubular secretion or active hepatic extraction will not be affected by changes in protein binding since such active processes can "strip" drug from protein sites, making both free and bound form are available for elimination.

Lidocaine is perhaps the most frequently administered anti-arrhythmic drug in the setting of acute MI. Many centers advocate its use prophylactically even before confirmation of infarct has been obtained (3). Because of its relatively narrow therapeutic range and the fact that it must be administered intravenously, the use of lidocaine is not without risk. In addition, there is evidence to suggest that lidocaine disposition in MI differs substantially from that in patients experiencing chest pain, but in whom there is no objective evidence of infarction (4). Lidocaine clearance correlates well with cardiac index (5). Myocardial infarction is often accompanied by diminished cardiac output, resulting in reduced hepatic blood flow and a smaller initial volume of distribution. These changes, in turn, result in a reduced clearance of lidocaine, which is principally eliminated by hepatic metabolism (6). Thus, the presence of cardiac failure will alter lidocaine kinetics. Administration of lidocaine to patients suspected of having MI results in a broad range of plasma levels (7), and there is accumulation of lidocaine in plasma during a constant infusion in those patients with confirmed MI (8,9,10). These observations are of interest both from a practical point of view in recommending dosage guidelines for lidocaine in patients with acute MI (11,12,13), and also in the determination of physiological processes responsible for these effects.

Zito and Reid (14) found a good correlation between the clearance of lidocaine and indocyanine green dye, and suggested a dosing regimen based on this relationship and the patients' degree of heart failure. However, Bax et al (15) could not confirm these findings in 17 post MI patients, although they did describe a more complex relationship between clearance of lidocaine and the reciprocal of indocyanine green half-life; the presence or absence of heart failure was of greater value in predicting lidocaine clearance (Figure 1).

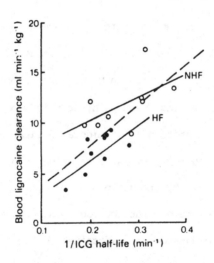

Figure 1. The relationship between the reciprocal of indocyanine green half-life and blood lidocaine clearances in patients without (O, NHF, n=9, y=22.18x + 5.75) and with (●, HF, n=9, y=37.0x - 0.87) heart failure, and in the group as a whole (broken line: n=18, y=39.85x - 0.27). From Reference 15, with permission.

Lopez et al (13) adopted the recommendations of Zito and Reid in 14 MI patients, comparing their plasma lidocaine levels to a control group of 18 MI patients who received a conventional dose of lidocaine. A narrower range of plasma concentrations and a significantly greater percentage of lidocaine levels within the accepted therapeutic range were noted in the experimental group compared to the control group. However, data were obtained for only five hours following the initiation of therapy, and no results regarding efficacy of the adjusted regimen were presented. This may be an important consideration, since many of the plasma levels of patients in the experimental group tended to be close to the lower end of the therapeutic range.

The elimination half-life of lidocaine is prolonged during long-term infusion following MI. In seven patients, three of whom had sustained an infarction, Bassan et al (16) reported a half-life of 90 min. after discontinuation of an 11-hour infusion. This value is not different from that found in normal subjects (17). However, after a long-term infusion (approximately 24 hours or more), in patients with MI, lidocaine elimination half-life has been reported in the 3-4 hour range (9,18), and, in one study, as long as 10 hours (10). Accompanying the increased elimination half-life is a rise in total plasma lidocaine concentration, and the time taken to reach steady state is prolonged. Based on a half-life of 90 min.in healthy subjects, one would expect steady-state to be achieved after approximately seven hours (17). However, in 12 patients with uncomplicated MI, who received a 1 mg/kg lidocaine bolus followed by an infusion at a rate of 20 mcg/kg/min, plasma concentration at 6-12 hours after the start of the infusion was 1.85+0.47 (mean+S.D.), compared to 4.32+1.64 at the end of the infusion lasting 25-60 hours (10). These data led the investigators to recommend that, after the first 24 hours the rate of infusion of lidocaine should be reduced by approximately one-half, even in patients without cardiac or hepatic failure, to compensate for the increased half-life and to avoid toxic plasma concentrations. Despite this potential for attainment of plasma levels exceeding the therapeutic range (2-6 mcg/mL), concentrations as high as 8 ug/ml have been reported to be well tolerated in some patients several days after MI (20).

Plasma protein binding may influence lidocaine kinetics shortly
after MI. Recently, Routledge et al (21) described a direct relationship between the plasma concentration of alpha –acid glycoprotein (AAG)$_1$
and the fraction of lidocaine bound. A rise in plasma AAG concentration
was accompanied by an increase in lidocaine binding and total plasma
lidocaine. The same group extended their observations to patients with
MI (20). AAG is an acute phase protein, whose concentration rises in
response to stress. Thus, in 15 patients with confirmed MI, AAG concentrations were significantly increased (117 mg/dL to 140 mg/dL) 36 hours
after infarction. There was no change in AAG concentration in 15 age
and sex matched control patients with chest pain only. In a more
detailed investigation of the relationship of AAG concentration and
lidocaine disposition, plasma lidocaine binding, total and free
lidocaine concentrations were measured over 12–48 hour after starting a
constant infusion (2 mg/min) in eight patients with confirmed MI, but
without heart failure or significant renal or hepatic disease (22). As
can be seen from Table 1, both total plasma lidocaine and AAG concentration rose progressively with time. The free lidocaine level,
however, remained fairly constant, so that the ratio of free/bound
fell. These observations help explain the rising total plasma levels of
lidocaine following MI, and, since the free, unbound drug is thought to
be the pharmacologically active moiety it may explain why total
lidocaine levels normally considered toxic can sometimes be tolerated
following acute MI. As a consequence, it also casts doubt on the
utility of total lidocaine plasma concentrations in guiding therapy in
this setting. One might also question the advice, based on total plasma
concentrations, to reduce the total lidocaine infusion rate by one-half
after 24 hours (10). This could bring the total concentration within

the usual therapeutic range, but might result in inadequate levels of free lidocaine in plasma, and presumably, at the effector sites.

Table 1. Effects of time on total and free plasma lidocaine concentrations, alpha-1-acid glycoprotein, and percent free lidocaine in eight patients with myocardial infarction on a constant 2 mg/min infusion (mean and range).

	Time (hours)			
	12	24	36	48
Total lidocaine (mcg/mL)	3.15 (1.9 - 4.1)	3.38 (1.7 - 4.5)	3.61 (1.6 -4.7)	4.23 ** (2.7 - 6.0)
Free lidocaine (mcg/mL)	0.99 (0.67-1.25)	0.99 (0.58-1.48)	1.02 (0.54-1.28)	1.11 (0.84-1.43)
AAG (mg/dL)	95 (57 - 127)	101 (61 - 137)	108 (78 - 136)	120 ** (91 - 152)
Free lidocaine (%)	0.31 (0.25-0.39)	0.30 (0.22-0.34)	0.29 (0.22-0.39)	0.27 * (0.21-0.32)

** p< 0.03 at 12, 24, and 36 hr.

* p< 0.05 at 12 and 24 hr.

From Reference 22, with permission.

In contrast to lidocaine, drug accumulation with prolonged infusion in acute MI has not been found with procainamide. Lalka et al (23) studied the kinetics of procainamide obtained during a 36-hour constant rate infusion in 5 MI patients; treatment was started 1-9 hours after onset of symptoms. Steady state was achieved between the 14th and 18th hour of infusion, which agrees well with data in volunteer studies. However, the plasma levels obtained in MI patients were markedly higher than would be predicted (Figure 2). These authors reported a reduced total body clearance of procainamide to about 60% of that in young healthy volunteers, although diminished renal function due to age differences may partially be responsible. In light of subsequent knowledge of increased binding of basic drugs in response to increased AAG in acute MI, the elevated plasma levels might also reflect increased protein binding.

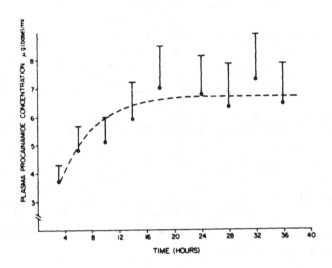

Figure 2. Mean plasma levels of procainamide (± 1 SEM) observed in five acute MI patients receiving a 3 mg/min constant-rate infusion of procainamide HCL (●); broken line is a simulation of a constant-rate infusion of 4.86 mg/min using average pharmacokinetic constants obtained from a large volunteer study. Note that volunteers would be expected to achieve a steady-state plasma concentration at nearly the same time as the patients were observed to have attained steady-state. However, 62% more drug would be required by the volunteers to maintain the same plasma concentration. From Reference 23, with permission.

Since AAG is a major binding protein for many basic drugs (24), other anti-arrhythmic agents such as disopyramide, propranolol and quinidine are also subject to changes in binding ratio as a result of increased AAG following MI.

Also of interest, in light of the altered kinetics of lidocaine in acute MI, are the observations with tocainide. This compound is structurally related to lidocaine, but is almost completely bioavailable after oral administration. In a study of tocainide kinetics in six healthy volunteers and sixteen patients with acute MI, Graffner et al (25) described similar kinetics in both groups of subjects. There were no differences between healthy subjects and patients with respect to elimination half-life (13.5 vs. 14.3 hours), apparent volume of distribution (2.9 vs. 3.2 L/kg) and total body clearance (2.6 mL/min kg), and patients' plasma levels remained within the therapeutic range during the study period; up to 168 hours.

That the pharmacokinetics of disopyramide are altered following MI has been recognized for some time. Ward and Kinghorn (26), using a variety of oral and intravenous regimens in patients within four hours of initial chest pain reported much lower disopyramide peak plasma concentrations and a decreased AUC compared to healthy volunteeers. In a study of seven patients receiving a single oral dose of disopyramide within 24 hours after the onset of infarction and again 7-14 days later, Jounela et al (27) also found lower peak serum concentration and a decreased bioavailability in the acute phase compared to convalescence (Figure 3). The 24-hour AUC was diminished and 48-hour urinary excretion of disopyramide was significantly less during the acute phase (29.6% of dose) than 7-14 days later (43.3% of dose). Both the 24-hour AUC and peak serum concentration showed a significant negative correlation with pulmonary capillary wedge pressure, suggesting that the bioavailability of disopyramide was inversely related to the degree of left ventricular failure. Elimination half-life and time-to-peak concentration were not different during the two phases. Other studies, however, have described delayed absorption and prolonged elimination half-life in confirmed infarct patients (28,29,30). Although the administration of narcotic analgesics is often suggested as responsible

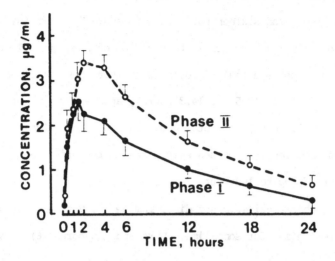

Figure 3. Mean ± SE serum levels of disopyramide obtained after administration of an oral dose of 200 mg disopyramide base to seven patients during the acute phase of myocardial infarction (phase I) and after recovery 7-14 days later (phase II). From Reference 27, with permission.

for delayed absorption, most studies have found a poor relationship between these factors (28,29). Great variability has been reported in elimination half-life, with values ranging from 7-38 hours (30,31) compared to a half-life of 6-8 hours in healthy volunteers. Some of the apparently divergent results may be explained by the timing of the study. Bryson et al (31) found no change in elimination half-life, absorption and bioavailability of disopyramide in nine patients, 3-14 days following infarction. They did ,however, describe a reduced volume of distribution and total clearance, similar to the changes repoted by Landmark (32) in patients with moderate cardiac failure.

Disopyramide elimination half-life is probably a reflection of its non-linear, dose-dependent plasma protein binding characteristics. As the total concentration of disopyramide increases, so does the free fraction (33). Meffin et al (34) calculated that a doubling of the total disopyramide concentration from 2 to 4 mg/L would result in a four-fold increase in free disopyramide concentration. A further complication is the increase in AAG concentration accompanying infarction. David et al (35) reported rising concentrations of AAG during the first five days following infarction, which had returned to initial levels at 3-20 weeks. The rise in AAG concentration was accompanied by a three-fold rise in the ratio of bound / free disopyramide.

Despite delayed absorption and low plasma levels accompanied by extensive protein binding, Kumana et al (29), in a study of 101 infarct patients, found prophylactic antiarrhythmic activity at disopyramide plasma levels (approximately 1.5 mg/L) below the normally accepted therapeutic range (2-4 mg/L).

Since MI is often accompanied by some degree of left ventricular failure, digitalis glycosides are often administered either for inotropic or anti-arrhythmic actions. Korhonen et al (36) compared the kinetics of a single dose of oral digoxin in 12 patients with left-heart failure due to MI and nine healthy volunteers. Although the absorption of digoxin was delayed in MI patients with significantly lower peak serum concentration (4.25 ± 0.59 ng/mL vs. 6.71 ± 0.41 ng/mL) and diminished 12 hour AUC, the total amount of digoxin absorbed as evidenced by 24-hour AUC and urinary excretion, did not differ. The 24 hour AUC was directly correlated to pulmonary capillary wedge pressure and heart rate, and both the digoxin renal clearance and urinary excretion correlated inversely with CK-MB (Figure 4) activity, suggesting that the severity of infarction may serve as a guide to changes in these pharmacokinetic variables.

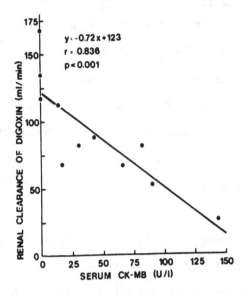

Figure 4. Renal clearance of digoxin diminished with CK-MB activity in 11 patients with infarction. U/l = units per liter. From Reference 36, with permission.

Prompted by the increasing use of intravenous beta blockade in the treatment of ischemic chest pain and arrhythmias, and possible utility in limiting infarct size (37), Vedin et al (38) investigated the pharmacokinetics of timolol in both healthy volunteers and patients with acute MI. They found no differences in elimination half-life, volume of distribution or plasma clearance between the two groups.

Acute MI also presents a particular problem in that the attendant arrhythmias probably arise from zones of ischemic myocardium (39). The heart is normally a highly perfused organ such that most anti-arrhythmic drugs in plasma rapidly equilibrate with myocardial tissue. In infarction, however, the very areas of poorly perfused myocardium which require anti-arrhythmic action may accumulate drug far more slowly than the rest of the heart. Delivery of lidocaine (40) and procainamide (41) to ischemic canine myocardium has been investigated.

Both studies showed a good direct relationship between regional myocardial blood flow and the time taken to reach steady state concentration. In the case of lidocaine, using a 24-hour-old infarct model, discrepancies in lidocaine concentration between normally-perfused and ischemic areas were evident within the first five minutes after bolus administration. In the case of procainamide, given as 5 X 1-minute infusions 5 minutes apart, within one hour of coronary artery ligation, a 16-fold difference in concentration between normally perfused and the most ischemic region existed at 5 minutes following drug infusion. After 25 minutes, procainamide concentration in the ischemic region was still only one third that in non-ischemic myocardium. Mildly ischemic areas reached steady-state concentration in 15-25 minutes. Figure 5 clearly illustrates the rapid rise and subsequent rapid decline of procainamide in non-ischemic tissue, compared to the attenuated rise and fall in progressively more ischemic areas, following a one-minute infusion of the drug.

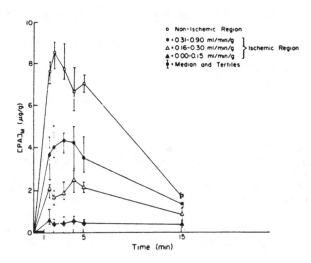

Figure 5. Myocardial procainamide concentrations plotted as a function of time following a one minute infusion of procainamide (horizontal bar). The data from ischemic sections were grouped by flow. Data are expressed as median and tertiles. From Reference 41, with permission.

From a practical point of view, extension of these observations to the clinical setting suggests that the temporal relationship between drug administration and effect may be altered in MI, since the poorly perfused areas of myocardium function as peripheral rather than central pharmacokinetic compartments.

Although each agent is unique in its pharmacokinetic profile, and dosing requirements in acute MI must often be determined empirically, several points should be borne in mind. Acute MI represents an unstable condition, often accompanied by decreased cardiac output. Blood flow to organs often important in the clearance of drugs is reduced, resulting in impaired renal or hepatic clearance. Heart failure reduces the initial volume of distribution. Half-life may often be prolonged. Changes in protein binding in response to increased AAG concentration can complicate the interpretation of total drug plasma level information.

Drugs likely to be administered in the acute phase of infarction should be evaluated in this setting, as routine extrapolation of data from healthy volunteers or patients with stable illness, to infarct patients, cannot be justified.

REFERENCES

1. Adgey AA, Allen JD, Geddes JS, James RGG, Webb SW, Zaidi SA, Pantridge JF: The acute phase of myocardial infarction. Lancet (ii): 501-504,1971.
2. Dhurandhar RW, MacMillan RL, Brown KWG: Primary ventricular fibrillation complicating acute myocardial infarction. Am J Cardiol (27): 347-351, 1971
3. Lie KI, Wellens HJ, Van Capelle FJ, Durrer D: Lidocaine in the prevention of primary ventricular fibrillation. N Engl J Med (291): 1324-1326, 1974
4. Barchowsky A, Shand DG, Stargel WW, Wagner GS, Routledge PA: On the role of alpha-1-acid glycoprotein in lignocaine accumulation following myocardial infarction. Br J Clin Pharmacol (13): 411-415, 1982

35

5. Thomson PD, Melmon KL, Richardson JA, Cohn K, Steinbrunn W, Cudihee R, Rowland M: Lidocaine pharmacokinetics in advanced heart failure, liver disease and renal failure in humans. Ann Intern Med (78): 499-508, 1973
6. Stenson RE, Constantino RT, Harrison DG: Inter-relationships of hepatic blood flow, cardiac output and blood levels of lidocaine in man. Circulation (43): 205-211, 1971
7. Zito RA, Reid PR, Longstreth JA: Variability of early lidocaine levels in patients. Am Heart J (94): 292-296, 1977
8. Aps C, Bell JA, Jenkins BS, Poole-Wilson PA, Reynolds F: Logical approach to lignocaine therapy. Br Med J (1): 13-15, 1976
9. Prescott LF, Adjepon-Yamoah KK, Talbot RG: Impaired lignocaine metabolism in patients with myocardial infarction and cardiac failure. Br Med J (1): 939-941, 1976
10. LeLorier J, Grenon D, Latour Y, Caille G, Dumont G, Brosseau A, Solignac A: Pharmacokinetics of lidocaine after prolonged infusions in uncomplicated myocardial infarction. Ann Intern Med (87): 700-702, 1977
11. Wyman MG, Lalka D, Hammersmith L, Cannom DS, Goldreyer BN: Multiple bolus technique for lidocaine administration during the first hours of an acute myocardial infarction. Am J Cardiol (41): 313-317, 1978
12. Hopperstead LO, Myers MH: Prophylactic lidocaine in the early management of acute myocardial infarction. J Maine Med Assoc (71):77-81, 1980
13. Lopez LM, Mehta JL, Robinson JD, Roberts RJ: Optimal lidocaine dosing in patients with myocardial infarction. Therap Drug Monit (4): 271-276, 1982
14. Zito RA, Reid PR: Lidocaine kinetics predicted by indocyanine green clearance. N Engl J Med (298): 1160-1163, 1978
15. Bax NDS, Tucker GT, Woods HF: Lignocaine and indocyanine green kinetics in patients following myocardial infarction. Br J Clin Pharmacol (10): 353-361, 1980
16. Bassan MM, Weinstein SR, Mandel WJ: Use of lidocaine by continuous infusion. Am Heart J (87): 302-303, 1974.
17. Boyes RN, Scott DB, Jebson PJ, Godman MJ, Julian DG: Pharmacokinetics of lidocaine in man. Clin Pharmacol Ther (12):105-116, 1971
18. Prescott LF, Nimmo J: Plasma lidocaine during and after prolonged infusion in patients with myocardial infarction. In: Scott DB, Julian DG (eds.) Lidocaine in the treatment of ventricular arrhythmias. Livingstone, Edinburgh, 1971, pp 168-177.
19. Hayes AH: Intravenous infusion of lidocaine in the control of ventricular arrhythmias. In: Scott DB, Julian DG (eds.) Lidocaine in the treatment of ventricular arrhythmias. Livingstone, Edinburgh, 1971, pp 189-199.
20. Routledge PA, Stargel WW, Wagner GS, Shand DG: Increased alpha-1-acid glycoprotein and lidocaine disposition in myocardial infarction. Ann Intern Med (93): 701-704, 1980
21. Routledge PA, Barchowsky A, Bjornsson TD, Kitchell BB, Shand DG: Lidocaine plasma protein binding. Clin Pharmacol Ther (27): 347-351, 1980
22. Routledge PA, Shand DG, Barchowsky A, Wagner G, Stargel WW: Relationship between alpha-1-acid glycoprotein and lidocaine disposition in myocardial infarction. Clin Pharmacol Ther (30): 154-157, 1981

23.   Lalka D, Wyman MG, Goldreyer BN, Ludden TM, Cannom DS: Procainamide accumulation kinetics in the immediate postmyocardial infarction period. J Clin Pharmacol (18): 397-401, 1978

24.   Piafsky KM: Disease-induced changes in the plasma binding of basic drugs. Clin Pharmacokinetics (5): 246-262, 1980

25.   Graffner C, Conradson TB, Hofvendahl S, Ryden L: Tocainide kinetics after intravenous and oral administration in healthy subjects and in patients with acute myocardial infarction. Clin Pharmacol Ther (27): 64-71, 1980

26.   Ward JW, Kinghorn GR: the pharmacokinetics of disopyramide following myocardial infarction with special reference to oral and intravenous dose regimens. J Int Med Res (4): Suppl. 1: 49-53, 1976

27.   Jounela AJ, Pentikainen PJ, Oksanen K: The pharmacokinetics of disopyramide in patients with acute myocardial infarction. Int J Clin Pharmacol Ther Toxicol (20): 276-282, 1982

28.   Weissberg PL, Matenga J, Hayler AM, Holt DW: Plasma disopyramide concentrations following a 300-mg oral loading dose in acute myocardial infarction. Therap Drug Monit (4): 277-280, 1982

29.   Kumana CR, Rambihar VS, Willis K, Gupta RN, Tanser PH, Cairns JA, Wildeman RA, Johnston M, Johnson AL, Gent M: Absorption and antidysrhythmic activity of oral disopyramide phosphate after acute myocardial infarction. Br J Clin Pharmacol (14): 529-537, 1982

30.   Ilett KF, Madsen BW, Woods JD: Disopyramide kinetics in patients with acute myocardial infarction. Clin Pharmacol Ther (26): 1-7, 1979

31.   Bryson SM, Cairns CJ, Whiting B: Disopyramide pharmacokinetics during recovery from myocardial infarction. Br J Clin Pharmacol (13): 417-421, 1982

32.   Landmark K, Bredesen JE, Thaulow E, Simonsen S, Amlie JP: Pharmacokinetics of disopyramide in patients with imminent to moderate cardiac failure. Eur J Clin Pharmacol (19): 187-192, 1981

33.   David BM, Madsen BW, Ilett KF: Plasma binding of disopyramide. Br J Clin Pharmacol (9): 614-618, 1980

34.   Meffin PJ, Robert EW, Winkle RA, Harapat S, Peters FA, Harrison DC: Role of concentration-dependent plasma protein binding in disopyramide disposition. J Pharmacokinetics Biopharmaceutics (7): 29-46, 1979

35.   David BM, Whitford EG, Ilett KF: Disopyramide binding to alpha-1-acid glycoprotein: sequential effects following acute myocardial infarction. Clin Exp Pharmacol Physiol (9):478, 1982

36.   Korhonen UR, Jounela AJ, Pakarinen AJ, Pentikainen PJ, Takkunen JT: Pharmacokinetics of digoxin in patients with acute myocardial infarction. Am J Cardiol (44): 1190-1194, 1979

37.   Peter T, Norris RM, Clarke ED, Heng MK, Singh BN, Williams B, Howell DR, Ambler PK: Reduction of enzyme levels by propranolol after acute myocardial infarction. Circulation (57): 1091-1095, 1978

38.   Vedin JA, Kristianson JK, Wilhelmsson CE: Pharmacokinetics of intravenous timolol in patients with acute myocardial infarction and in healthy volunteers. Eur J Clin Pharmacol (23): 43-47, 1982.

39. Waldo AL, Kaiser GA: A study of ventricular arrhythmias associated with acute myocardial infarction in the canine heart. Circulation (47): 1222-1228, 1973

40.   Zito RA, Caride VJ, Holford T, Zaret BL: Regional myocardial kinetics of lidocaine in experimental infarction: modulation by regional blood flow. Am J Cardiol (47): 265-270, 1981

41.   Wenger TL, Browning DJ, Masterton CE, Abou-Donia MB, Harrell FE Jr, Bache RJ, Strauss HC: Procainamide delivery to ischemic canine myocardium following rapid intravenous administration. Circ Res (46): 789-795, 1980

4

LIMITATIONS OF ELECTROPHYSIOLOGIC TECHNIQUES IN DEFINING MYOCARDIAL
INFARCT SIZE

E. Neil Moore and Joseph F. Spear, University of Pennsylvania, School of
Veterinary Medicine, Philadelphia, Pa.

Electrophysiologists are usually more concerned with the heart's
ability to generate action potentials than its ability to be an efficient
pump. Of course, even electrophysiologists have to admit that the primary
function of the heart is to be an efficient dependable blood pump. It has
been known for many years that electrical activity of the heart can
appear reasonably normal at a time when the contractability of the art is
rapidly deteriorating. In order for the heart to be an efficient pump, it
is necessary that the cardiac cells be activated in their normal, orderly
sequence of activation during each cardiac cycle and that each cardiac cell
is capable of delivering its share towards mechanical contractility. At the
time of a myocardial infarction, determining the size of the myocardial
infarct, as well as being able to measure any subsequent changes in size of
the infarct is necessary both to permit optimal treatment of the patient as
well as to determine whether various treatments are actually increasing the
number and improving the function of cardiac cells that are saved from cell
death.

It is important to know how accurately electrophysiological
techniques can distinguish and quantify myocardial tissue that is
irreversibly damaged from that which is normal or reversibly injured. There
are basically three major techniques that are available to the
electrophysiologist for assessing electrical activity of the heart. The
most ideal noninvasive techniques are electrocardiographic methods where the
electrical activity of the heart is analyzed via electrodes located at
different places on the body. The second electrophysiologic technique is to
record cardiac electrograms directly from a group of cardiac cells, either
at the time of cardiac surgery or via recording catheters introduced at the
time of cardiac catheterization. The third electrophysiological method
employs ultramicroelectrodes to record the transmembrane electrical activity
of single cardiac cells. The ability and limitations of these three

electrophysiological techniques to indicate cardiac cell function and cell damage will be discussed under three major headings: 1) electrocardiographic methods , 2) direct cardiac electrogram recording methods and 3) cellular cardiac electrophysiological methods.

Electrocardiographic Methods

The ideal method for measuring infarct size would be an electrocardiographic method. The advantage of an electrocardiographic method is that electrocardiograms are routinely available and can be obtained in a non-invasive manner. Unlike many other methods such as radionucleotides and positron tomography techniques, the electrocardiogram is also a very economical way to evaluate infarct size. In addition, repeat measurements can be made at short intervals and it is not necessary to wait many hours for outprinting of results. However, with a standard 12-lead electrocardiogram, it is usually not possible to accurately distinguish in any quantitative fashion what the precise size of the infarct is. One can distinguish a small from a massive or moderate size infarct, but with electrocardiographic methods it is difficult to predict even 5 to 10% changes in the ventricular mass. Numerous investigators have tried computer processing of electrocardiograms in order to see if additional information can be obtained. Of course one advantage of the electrocardiogram being computer analyzed is that the same computer programs can be used in the community hospital as well as in the university setting.

One reason that the electrocardiogram has great limitations in its ability to predict the size of an infarct has been pointed out by Abildskov (1). He states that at least 80% of the ventricular mass is normally excited in such a manner that vectorcardiographic effects are cancelled. Therefore one is limited to only 20% of the information concerning cardiac electrical activation being available on the body's torso. This certainly provides sufficient information to indicate whether one has a massive or small infarct, and also permits estimation of the region where the infarct has occurred. However, if one is giving a drug or utilizing some method to try to save ischemic cells, then standard electrocardiographic methodologies have very definite limitations in indicating small changes in the number of viable versus non-viable cardiac cells.

With the development of larger computers, renewed efforts have been made to obtain the maximal amount of information from the ECG concerning cardiac activation and function. Approaches have included computer modeling techniques as well as techniques recording multiple arrays of precordial electrocardiograms for computer quantification. Of course electrocardiograms recorded from multiple sites contain duplicate as well as unique information concerning cardiac activation. The ability of a computer to analyze great quantities of data, to filter out the unique from repetitious information and to provide this information in a reasonably short period of time has encouraged numerous electrocardiographic approaches to quantifying infarcts. One interesting method is departure mapping which has been suggested and utilized by Flowers and associates (2). Departure mapping consists of establishing a data bank of statistically normal precordial electrocardiograms recorded at multiple thoracic sites and then comparing the electrocardiogram in a patient having cardiac disease with these statistically normal electrogram using computer assisted subtraction methods. The display of the difference between what normally should be recorded at that precordial site versus the electrocardiogram actually recorded is the departure signal. A departure map contains not only the information at a single site, but sums all precordial map sites in order to get an estimation of abnormalities in cardiac activation. However, departure maps may be difficult to interpret during ischemic injury and infarction since the extracellular recorded potentials are influenced by alteration both in spatial and in non-spatial factors during ischemia injury and infarction. Nevertheless, departure ECG mapping is an exciting new approach which is idea for computer automation and which provides a resulting departure electrocardiogram that most cardiologists can readily understand due to its similarity to normally recorded ECG's.

A second electrocardiographic method for estimating the distribution of myocardial potentials on the body surface is inverse mapping. Barr and Spach recently used this technique in an attempt to predict what the myocardial potentials on the epicardial surface should be based on the recorded precordial electrocardiogram (3). The inverse mapping technique is compromised both by the problem of the loss of electrophysiologic information from the myocardium as well as modification of the electrical signals by the non-linear transfer function of the human torso. Despite these limitations they found that they could obtain the general features of epicardial depolarization and repolarization. Although considerable refinement of this technique is still necessary before it can be useful in predicting infarct size it may nevertheless allow us to select the precordial sites which provide the greatest amount of information concerning myocardial activation based on ECG recordings on the body torso.

A third ECG technique for estimating infarct size is the QRST area map technique. Recently Abildskov's group has found in experimental studies in dogs, that the QRST area maps may actually reflect changes in refractory periods at different sites and are largely independent of activation sequence (4). If this turns out to be true, then it may be possible to obtain an indication of the disparity in recovery properties of the heart in different locations. It is well known that the greater the disparities in refractory periods are the greater is the tendency of the heart to develop lethal tachyarrhythmias.

A fourth approach to improving electrocardiographic methods for predicting infarct size is the computer modeling approach of Selvester and his colleagues (5). Selvester first cross-sectioned a normal heart and then using inline digitizing tables introduced the complex anatomical geometries of the heart into a computer model. In this way specification of the size and location of papillary muscles, ventricular wall thickness and local variations in regional wall geometry could be included. Selvester next introduced into the model the different activation times for the respective digitized anatomical regions the electrical activation studies of Durer (6) and Scher (7). The pathway of ventricular depolarizaton was simulated using special numerical methods of wavefront construction for a three dimensional region and thus the model can predict the activation sequence of the heart. The model also transfers the electrical analogs of local myocardial activation to the body surface and even introduces the effects of the inhomogeneous bounded torso volume conductor properties of the body. With this model using a normal male torso geometry and resistivities they have analyzed the effects of ventricular enlargement, conduction abnormalities and localized myocardial infarcts. These experiments have allowed them to analyze the effects on the inscribed electrocardiograms of very small infarcts at different locations within the various coronary vessel's distribution. In this way they have determined what the electrocardiographic effects would be with a single pure infarct, for example the proximal 5 mm of the left anterior descending coronary artery. They also have analyzed the effects of complicating ventricular hypertrophy, conduction abnormalities and prior infarction (loss of activity) in other regions. Using this computer simulation model they have now developed a point system which allows them to predict the effect on the ECG of a loss of each 3% increment of the left ventricular mass. Modeling is a very exciting approach to understanding electrocardiographic recordings. The complexities of differing heart geometry as well as the complexities of disease processes resulting in hypertrophy, conduction defects and myocardial abnormalities are now being investigated. This ECG model should allow at least the estimation of what is the maximum amount of information available in the ECG for predicting infarct size. The cost and repeatability of easily taking electrocardiograms at multiple times certainly makes the effort to develop an accurate electrocardiographic method for depicting infarct size an important area of research.

Direct Cardiac Electrograms - Ability to Predict Infarct Size.

Cardiac electrograms can be recorded directly from multiple sites on the endocardial surface of the heart at the time of cardiac catheterization. In addition electrograms can be recorded from most any epicardial or transmural site of the heart at the time of open heart surgery. Unfortunately even recording directly from infarcted sites and normal sites can pose difficulties in predicting the degree of myocardial damage. For example, early electrogram recordings may suggest that the ischemic cells are irreversibly damaged yet, with reperfusion these cells may recover normal excitability. As Reimer has pointed out elsewhere in this monograph, total irreversible cardiac cell death often does not occur until nearly three hours of continual ischemia. Rapid intrinsicoid triphasic potentials are usually recorded from normal tissue while from an infarct one records low amplitude long duration potentials. These low amplitude long duration potentials may actually represent nothing more than electrotonically conducted distant electrical activity from surrounding cardiac fibers, i.e. the cells underneath the electrode may be totally dead. At the border of infarcted and normal tissue, multiphasic electrograms are often recorded. Thus it is very difficult to quantitatively describe the region of damage using epicardial and/or endocardial mapping electrodes since the electrogram recorded depends very much on the dimension of the electrode, the electrode-tissue interface and even still more upon the geometry of the infarct. A heterogeneous "swiss-cheese" type infarct can present very long duration multiple fast spike electrograms while a homogeneous dense scarred infarct usually has long duration low amplitude electrograms. The use of multipolar electrode needles similar to those used by Boineau when placed through the myocardial wall probably provides as accurate an electrophysiological way of identifying infarct dimensions as is presently available (8). However, these small 22 gauge needles with 15 recording points located at 1 mm intervals, provides so much data that the analysis becomes very unwieldy unless a large computer is available to handle the data. Thus while it is possible using multipolar intramural electrodes to estimate the geometry of the infarct, the procedure requires a thoracotomy and the data is never available immediately. This limits the usefulness of the technique for analyzing treatments aimed at modifying infarct size.

The use of multipolar catheters for recording electrical activity to define infarct size and location is fraught with numerous difficulties. It is never a certainty of exactly where the catheter is located, nor can one even be certain of how large an area of the heart that the cathode records electrical activity from. For example, the circular electrodes on the catheter records from both the cavity of the ventricle as well as from that part of the circle electrode which is in apposition with the ventricular myocardium. In fact a recording catheter can even not be in apposition with the ventricular wall and still record a larger electrogram than is possible if one has a discrete bipolar electrode in direct apposition with the ventricular wall. In figure 1 a small discrete electrode and a catheter electrode are located on the surface of the myocardium and then are step-wise lifted off the surface and the different distances measured by a micrometer. It can be noted that the amplitude of the potential recorded with the discrete electrodes falls off very rapidly with distance away from the tissue while the circular catheter electrodes continues to record substantial electrical activity as the electrodes are removed from the myocardial surface. This emphasizes the importance of electrode configuration and the difficulties of identifying the precise region where one is recording with catheters. Further difficulties in recording with catheter electrodes results from the fact that frequently although one records bipolarly with a catheter, actually only one pole is in proximity

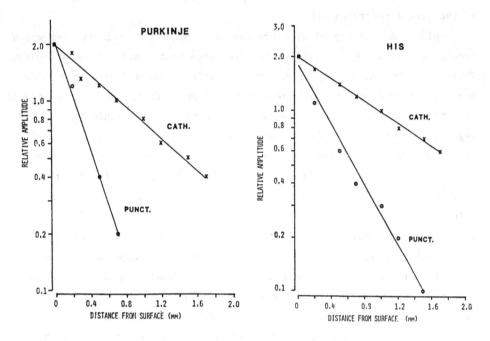

FIGURE 1

In A, the relative amplitude of a Purkinje fiber electrogram versus
distance from the surface of the Purkinje fiber is shown. Electrograms were
recorded with either a bipolar punctate electrode (Punct.) or with a bipolar
recording catheter (Cath.). It can be noted that the amplitude of the
recorded Purkinje fiber electrogram decreased much more rapidly as the
punctate electrode was lifted off the surface of the tissue than occurred
with the catheter recording electrodes. The canine Purkinje fiber was
superfused with Tyrode's solution and pinned to the bottom of an isolated
tissue chamber.

In B, similar electrogram amplitude measurements were made in an
isolated canine bundle of His preparation as a punctate bipolar electrode
(Punct.) and a bipolar catheter electrode (Cath.) were lifted stepwise off
the surface of the preparation. Again, the amplitude of the bundle of His
electrogram as recorded by the punctate electrode decrease more rapidly with
distance from the surface of the preparation than occurred with the bipolar
catheter electrode. These findings emphasize the problems of knowing the
precise region from which an electrode records electrical activity.

44

with the tissue and it is only that single pole of the bipolar catheter that records electrical activity. Thus activity may be recorded either at the distal or proximal electrode and depending upon the relative distance between the electrodes, one can be considerably off in estimating location of the actual recording site.

Epicardial mapping of ST elevation as a measure of infarct size was a technique that enjoyed considerable acceptance in the mid and early 1970's. There is no question that ST segment elevation appears following coronary occlusion in regions that are infarcted. However, there can be considerable variability in ST elevation when measured site-to-site within the infarct region, and time lapse following infarctions affects the recorded ST elevation magnitude. Simson pointed out that if one measures the average ST elevation at the border of the infarct to normal tissue and takes that as representative of dead tissue, then one can find that up to 81% of the epicardial region overlying the infarct will be measured as having lower ST elevations than that region (9). In Simson's studies they determined the normal-infarct junction using an NADH flourescent technique which precisely identified normal from abnormal tissues. This finding by Simson was also supported by the studies from Irvin and Cobb (10) who found a very poor correlation between histologic necrosis and ST segment elevation. The reason for the wide variation in ST elevation with infarction has been nicely described in a review by Holland and Arnsdorf (11). They analyzed the effects of location and shape of the ischemic area on the solid angle from which the electrode would record. They demonstrated that subepicardial infarcts would result in outward current flow from normal tissue into the subepicardial infarct whereas with a subendocardial infarct, current flow during the ST segment would be in the opposite direction from the outer normal epicardial region into the infarcted subendocardial region. If the infarct becomes transmural, then current flows are even more complicated. When one deals with even more complicated geometry of the infarct such as in the chronic canine ischemia model where a mottled "swiss-cheese" type infarct occurs, then one can easily understand the difficulties for any extracellular potential recording technique to define precisely the percent or region of myocardium damaged.

It is quite clear that more sophisticated electrophysiological studies are needed in order to make adequate quantification of infarct size and to allow analysis of the effects of boundaries surrounding the

evolving infarct and the extracellularly recorded potentials. It is clear
that we need to be able to use extracellular recorded signals to predict
tissue viability and death. To do this will require new techniques to allow
us to recover more information about the underlying electrophysiological
events then we presently have.

Intracellular Methods for Estimating Infarct Size

It is possible to remove tissues containing the area of infarct and
to record intracellular action potentials from the isolated preparation.
Clearly one can identify normal cells from dead cells. However, geometrical
complexity can result in some membrane potentials being lower than normal
and action potential amplitudes and configuration altered from normal due to
the electrotonic interactions between adjacent normal and abnormal fibers.
The complicated coupling and uncoupling that develops between normal,
abnormal and dead cells is difficult to analyze even with microelectrode
techniques. Also, with microelectrodes one can only record 4 or 5 cell
layers deep and thus it is impossible to obtain a three dimensional map of
an infarct using the microelectrode technique. In order to accurately
analyze and predict extracellular recorded potentials, we need to develop
ways to identify what is going on in deeper layers. Microelectrode
studies are lacking to explain the complexities that actually exist in an
infarct as to current flows during activation and recovery, i.e. the
inscription of the QRS, the ST and TQ intervals.

Future Directions: Low Level Body Surface Potentials

Unfortunately electrophysiological techniques are presently unable to
precisely identify irreversibly injured cells from those which are normal
and reversibly injured. It is known that in regions where lethal
tachyarrhythmias develop that reentry frequently is present. and that
reentry can be associated with continuous rapid deflections that persist
into the ST interval. A new electrophysiological technique that has shown
great promise for identifying hearts having electrical instability is high
gain signal averaged, digitally filtered electrocardiograms in which low
level body surface electrical activity persisting into the ST time interval
is evaluated (12). Any persistent low level deflections in the high gain
signal averaged ECG signify a potential for arrhythmogenesis. This
signal averaged technique is one that is receiving considerable attention as

a non-invasive technique for identifying hearts with electrical instability
and a tendency for developing lethal arrhythmias.

Summary

In summary, although great efforts are being made to evaluate and
limit the size of an infarct, it also must be remembered that even small
infarcts can result in lethal arrhythmias. Most of the patients who
experience sudden cardiac death do so because their hearts become
electrically unstable and ventricular fibrillation occurs. In our efforts
to decrease the size of myocardial infarcts we must not reduce infarct
size at the expense of creating more electrically unstable hearts. In
fact, if one causes a mottled "swiss-cheese" type infarct with
interspersing of normal and abnormal tissues as a result of treatment of
myocardial ischemia, then the heart actually may have a higher propensity to
developing lethal arrhythmias despite the fact that fewer cardiac cells
died. On the other hand, a more homogeneous infarct seems to have less
tendency for developing ventricular fibrillation and sudden death.

We now have the ability to use sophisticated computer assisted
techniques to look at the small amount of information that is not
cancelled out in the activation process of the heart. Hopefully we will
be able to develop techniques to obtain maximal information from this
electrical activity that will allow us to not only predict hearts with
good electrical stability and decreased tendency for developing lethal
arrhythmias but also to be able to identify in a more quantitative manner
the size of the myocardial infarct. By identifying the size of an
infarct, we can then judge whether our treatment is being successful or
unsuccessful and better direct our therapy for treatment of myocardial
infarction.

Acknowledgements: We thank the W.W. Smith Charitable Trust and the National
Heart, Lung and Blood Institute for support and Bejay Moore for typing the
manuscript.

Bibliography

1. Abildskov, J.A.: The relation of localized myocardial lesion size to the QRS complex of vector cardiographic leads. J. Electrocardiography 13:(4), 307-310, 1980.

2. Flowers, N.C., Horan, L.G., Sohi G.S., Hand, R.C., Johnson, J.C.: New evidence for inferoposterior myocardial infarction on surface potential maps. Am. J. Cardiol. 38:576, 1976.

3. Spach, M.S., Barr, R.C., Warren, R.B., Benson, D.W., Walston, A, Edwards, S.B.: Isopotential body surface mapping in subjects of all ages: emphasis on low-level potentials with analysis of the method. Circulation 59:805-821, 1979.

4. Abildskov, J.A., Evans, A.K., Lux, R.L., Burgess, M.J.: Direct evidence relating QRST deflection area and ventrticular recovery properties (abstr.) Circulation 60 (Suppl 2): 11-110, 1979.

5. Selvester, R.H., Sanmarco, M.E., Solomon, J.C. and Wagner, G.S.: The ECG: QRS Change. In: Wagner, G.S. (ed.) Myocardial Infarction: Measurement and Intervention, pp. 23-50. Martinus Nijhoff Publishers, The Hague/Boston/London 1982.

6. Durrer, D., vanDam, R.T., Meijler F.L., Arzbaecher, R.C., Mueller, E.J., Freud G.E.: Electrical activation and membrane action potentials of a perfused, normal heart (abstr.) Circulation 34:III-92, 1966.

7. Scher, A.M. and Young, A.C.: The pathway of ventricular depolarization in the dog. Circ. Res. 4:461, 1956.

8. Boineau , J.P., Hill, J.D., Spach, M.S. and Moore, E.N. Basis of the ECG in right ventricular hypertrophy: correlation of ventricular and body surface potentials during QRS and ST in dogs with spontaneous RVH. Am. Heart J. 76:605, 1968.

9. Simson, M.B., Harden, W.R., Barlow, C.H. and Harken, A.H.: Epicardial ischemia as delineated with epicardial ST segment mapping and nicotinamide adenine dinucleotide (NADH) flourescent photography. Am. J. Cardiol. 44: 263-269, 1979.

10. Irvin R.G. and Cobb, F.R.: Relationship between epicardial ST-segment elevation , regional myocardial blood flow and extent of myocardial infarction in awake dogs. Circulation 55:825-832, 1977.

11. Arnsdorf, M.F. and Louie, E.K.: The ECG: The spatial and nonspatial determinants of the extracellularly recorded potential with emphasis on the TQ-ST segment. In: Wagner, G.S. (ed). Myocardial Infarction: Measurement and Intervention, pp. 51-106, Martinus Nijhoff Publishers, The Hague/Boston/London, 1982.

12. Simson, M.B. : Use of signals in the terminal QRS complex to identify patients with ventricular tachycardia after myocardial infarction. Circ. 64:235-242, 1981.

5

ESTIMATES OF INJURY AFTER INFARCTION EVOLVING SPONTANEOUSLY OR IN RESPONSE TO
CORONARY THROMBOLYSIS

Dr. Burton Sobel

An early impetus for measuring infarct size was the need to determine
whether it presaged long-term prognosis. Patients with small infarcts measured
with the enzymatic method developed in our laboratory in the 1970's were
found, in fact, to exhibit better long-term prognosis than those with larger
infarcts based on life-table analysis. It is, of course, obvious that the
extent of infarction may not be the cause of the difference. The difference
could be due to the severity of underlying vascular disease or a host of other
factors. Nevertheless, it seems sensible to conclude that a small infarct is
less undesirable than a large one.

The impetus was intensified by Rentrop's pioneering treatment of
infarction with thrombolytic therapy. His work demonstrated unequivocally
that activators of the thrombolytic system given systemically or via the
coronary arteries could lyse clots.

It was soon clear that thrombolytic therapy was promising, as had been
presaged by results of others obtained in the mid-1970's.

How can we properly and definitively assess such therapy? Clots can be
lysed. That has been demonstrated unequivocally. The crucial question is
however, "What happens to the patient in the long term?" We do not yet know
what the impact of clot lysis will be on the heart itself, let alone on the
patient. Does lysis change the amount of apparent tissue injury, modify
electrical instability, or improve ventricular performance? These endpoints
may be distorted profoundly by the intervention itself. It is well
appreciated, for example, that reperfusion alters evolution of the
electrocardiographic changes with respect to what would have been observed if
the infarct had proceeded along its usual course. How to interpret these
changes is moot.

Results by Anderson and others demonstrate that streptokinase alters the
shape of the plasma enzyme time-activity curve. The message is, however,

complex. Does the change mean that more enzyme was liberated from the heart when streptokinase was given than would have been the case if the patient had experienced a spontaneously evolving infarction? Conversely, does the area under the curve exceed what it would have been in the absence of thrombolysis? Doe we simply visualize increased washout of enzyme that occurs at a faster rate without an augmentation of the overall amount released? If so, can we use conventional plasma CK methods of analysis for quantification of infarction in the face of reperfusion? If there is a difference in the total amount of enzyme released, the integrated area under the curve would be larger. Is it? If so, does that imply a larger infarct? Did streptokinase in fact make the infarct worse? Or does the observation mean that more enzyme was released into the circulation that would have been otherwise because of a decrease in the amount destroyed locally within the heart. The answers to these and related questions are not yet available. Evangelical spokesmen abound on both sides in each of the issues, but conclusions are not yet clear.

In experimental animals, plasma CK curves continue to faithfully represent infarct size despite reperfusion after 4 hr or more. However, earlier reperfusion results in a relatively larger amount of enzyme being released into the circulation than would have been the case with the same extent of infarction in the absence of reperfusion. In other words, distortion of the curve reflects a larger amount of enzyme released per gram of myocardium undergoing necrosis. Thus, interpretation of enzyme data depends on the time of onset of reperfusion with respect to the time of onset of ischemia (1).

Some information is available that sheds light on some of these issues. Measurements of the myocardial CK release-depletion ratio which reflects the proportion of enzyme lost from the heart that enters the circulating blood provides some insight. With reperfusion in dogs subjected to ischemia for 4 to 6 hr, the ratio is the same as that seen after fixed occlusion. However, with reperfusion implemented 40 to 120 min after the onset of ischemia, approximately twice as much enzyme enters the circulating blood compared with the amount that would have entered the circulation with an infarct of comparable extent in the absence of reperfusion (1).

In the late 1970's, Wevers and others made a very interesting observation. Chromatograms performed with agarose exhibited shoulders in the MM CK isoenzyme peak ultimately shown to reflect subforms of the individual MM

CK isoenzyme (2). We recently expanded on these observations, first by employing a method that had been developed in San Francisco by Drs. Morelli and Rapaport and colleagues employing isoelectric focusing (3) and subsequently with a chromatofocusing procedure which we developed to avoid denaturation of subforms of individual isoenzymes of CK (isoforms) and improve their differentiation (4). Chromatofocusing of MM isoenzyme purified from heart muscle yields a single, clean peak. However, when enzyme from this peak (MM_A) is incubated in plasma, in the test tube, or in the circulation, additional peaks (MM_B and MM_C) appear reflecting conversion of MM_A to subforms with the same antigenic properties and the same specific enzymatic activity. Conversion appears to be mediated by a factor in plasma in saturating concentrations since it occurs at a constant rate in experimental animals and patients. The chemistry has not yet been worked out in detail but the bold strokes are clear. The fractions of MM_A in blood, the parent form which is presumably the gene product in the myocardium, declines monoexponentially in vitro or in vivo. The decline of MM_A as a percentage of total MM activity is associated with simultaneous appearance of MM_B and subsequently MM_C. We have recently found that conversion is sequential with MM_A yielding only MM_B and MM_B yielding only MM_C. None of these steps is reversible. Thus, we have a convenient, biological clock. Since conversion occurs only after the enzyme has been released from the heart into plasma, the ratios of subforms in a blood sample and the rate of change of the ratio in serial samples define the age of the infarct. This phenomenon permits resolution of some of the interpretative questions related to washout and the effect of thrombolytic therapy. A large MM_A fraction in a sample obtained 2 hr after the apparent onset of pain does not reflect an infarct of the same overall magnitude as would be the case if the same total enzyme activity were constituted by the usually seen ratio of MM_B to MM_A. Instead, the enzyme elevation can be attributed, in part, to increased net washout with insufficient time for conversion of MM_A to MM_C in the circulation.

Ventricular function has been taken to be a useful criterion in assessing the efficacy of coronary thrombolysis. However, we and others have seen several examples of patients undergoing angiographically documented successful reperfusion to manifest no improvement in ventricular performance judging from overall ejection fraction or regional wall motion abnormalities (5). The lack of improvement may reflect an infarct of relatively advanced age among a host of possible explanations. On the other hand, ventricular function sometimes improves persistently despite reocclusion after transiently successful clot lysis. Although the paradox may be due to changes in collateral blood flow or other factors, it is clear that ventricular function does not bear a direct relation to the efficacy of reperfusion.

Many years ago Willerson and co-workers demonstrated convincingly that the "no reflow" phenomenon occurred in the heart. Thus, myocardial perfusion after relief of coronary obstruction in place for several hours is accompanied by very early reflow that does not persist or by limited initial reflow despite restoration of vascular patency. Compromise in nutritional flow may be due to capillary endothelial swelling, hemorrhage into the heart, or intracardiac edema. Regardless of its cause, the status of the nutritional blood flow cannot be predicted simply from the coronary angiogram.

For these and related reasons, we have been working since the mid-1970's on methods of measuring myocardial blood flow and myocardial metabolism quantitatively in man with a noninvasive approach applicable to research in this area. Our approach involves positron emission tomography (PET) (6-10). It exploits the physical properties of tracers labeled with positron-emitting radionuclides that permit quantification of their distribution in a fashion very analogous to that used for quantification in CT scanning. The physics are such that one can reconstruct the distribution of tracers in quantitative terms as opposed to the case with single photon emitting tracers assessed with a conventional camera system in which quantification can never be ideal. We have used PET with carbon-11 labeled palmitate (^{11}C-palmitate), a counterpart of the physiological substrate of the heart, to define regional metabolism and with water labeled with oxygen-15 ($H_2^{15}O$) to define regional myocardial blood flow. Extensive work in the experimental animal laboratory has documented the extent to which the measurements are valid (6-12).

Recently, we have applied this approach to assessing thrombolytic therapy. In experimental animals we induced coronary thrombi with a copper coil tipped coronary arterial catheter. Complete occlusion occurs within 30 min heralded by reperfusion arrhythmia and the electrocardiographic signs of incipient and evolving infarction. With thrombolytic therapy, clot lysis occurs promptly though the coil is of course still in place. Electrocardiographic changes evolve just as they do in patients. The tomograms delineate effects of the intervention on the heart. As shown in Figure 1, impaired metabolism is ameliorated substantially by thrombolysis. Thus, clot lysis initiated early after the onset of ischemia can restore regional myocardial metabolism in cells that have remained viable during the antecedent interval of ischemia (13).

On the other hand, not all examples are so gratifying. In some dogs no change occurred in the tomograms even though clot lysis was induced and vascular patency was restored. When ischemia was present for several hours, metabolism generally did not improve. The clinical implications are obvious. If thrombolytic therapy can do harm, and we believe that it can at least under some circumstances, it should not be employed with abandon or under conditions in which myocardial viability is so compromised in the cells within the region of supply of the occluded vessel that restoration of blood flow offers no hope of restoration of regional myocardial survival. There should be at least reasonable expectation that the myocardium within the zone of supply of the occluded vessel is capable of responding to reperfusion. Figure 2 illustrates the time-dependence in animals subjected to occlusion and reperfusion induced with streptokinase after ischemia of selected intervals induced by imposition of coronary thrombosis. Improvement of metabolism accompanies reperfusion implemented early, but not reperfusion delayed for 4 to 6 hr or more.

What about perfusion? After administration of labeled water intravenously, wash-in to myocardium is proportional to flow. In order to measure wash-in, Drs. Bergmann and Fox in our laboratory developed a method for subtracing the $H_2{}^{15}O$, is administered by inhalation. It binds to hemoglobin. The ratio of $H_2{}^{15}O$ to C^{15} can be determined within the vascular pool from tomograms delineating the intracavitary radioactivity within the left ventricle. Myocardial perfusion can be calculated by correcting myocardial $H_2{}^{15}O$ activity for activity of $H_2{}^{15}O$ within the same field of view but attributable to $H_2{}^{15}O$ in the blood pool. The factor required for this calculation is the $C^{15}O$ activity within the same field of view of myocardium. Results have been validated with gallium-labeled microspheres (12).

In experimental animals and patients, tomography provides comparable information. When reperfusion is implemented relatively late, flow increases, but metabolism is not restored. Thus, time is an absolutely critical parameter for salutary effects of thrombolysis on the heart (14).

Streptokinase is clearly not an ideal activator of the fibrinolytic system for clinical use. In essence, when we use it or urokinase to induce fibrinolysis, we convert plasminogen, a zymogen in the blood, to plasmin yielding a circulating proteolytic enzyme that non-specifically destroys other circulating proteins. It will lyse clots, but it will also degrade numerous essential moieties in the blood such as fibrinogen which is then depleted from the circulation. As a result of this very non-specific action, systemic bleeding is potentiated. The extent of the bleeding tendency is somewhat controversial, but several reports attest to an incidence as high as 10 to 44%. Although the phenomenon is somewhat dose-related, it is not readily controllable. For intravenous use such activators must be given in higher concentrations that is the case for intracoronary use. Accordingly, the bleeding risk is intensified (5,15).

Over the past several years, we have been studying activators that do not produce plasmin in the circulating blood. Some are called tissue-type plasminogen activators or vascular activators. These agents have the unique property of expressing their biological activity essentially only when bound to fibrin. In the absence of clot, the activator "can't find" the plasminogen in the blood because its affinity for circulating plasminogen is so low. With clot present, the activator binds to fibrin and the complex exhibits a very high affinity for plasminogen which also binds to fibrin in small quantities. Plasmin is generated at the fibrin surface of the clot but not in the circulating blood. Thus, fibrinogen is not depleted, circulating plasminogen is not depleted, $alpha_2$-antiplasmin is not consumed and fibrinogen degradation products do not accumlate. A bleeding diathesis is therefore not induced. These features contrast with the case with streptokinase or urokinase (6).

Many patients with myocardial infarction will require surgery early after the onset of their acute episode or percutaneous transluminal coronary angioplasty (PTCA) to definitively correct high grade, residual stenosis. Some will require cardiac catheterization. All are subject to some unavoidable trauma in the hospital. Thus, bleed tendencies must be minimized.

In our initial studies, a human tissue-type plasminogen activator (t-PA) was isolated and purified in a cell culture system and given intravenously to dogs with induced coronary thrombi. Reperfusion was prompt (often with 10 min). PET with $H_2^{15}O$ and ^{11}C-palmitate demonstrated improved perfusion and improved myocardial metabolism (Figure 3). However, systemic activation of the fibrinolytic system did not occur in contrast to the case with streptokinase (16). Preliminary results in patients are similar.

The conclusions are straightforward. Assessment of thrombolysis requires endpoints on its effects on the heart that are not distorted by the intervention itself. Conventionally used endpoints of infarction must be reexamined in terms of the questions we all seek to resolve in the years to come. Fortunately, new information such as that relating to conversion of isoforms of individual isoenzymes should serve to clarify interpretation of data acquired in the setting of coronary thrombolysis. The likely availability of activators of the fibrinolytic system already demonstrated to be devoid of the risk of induction of systemic bleeding makes thrombolytic therapy particularly attractive. Positron emission tomography appears to offer particular promise of answering the important question of what such therapy does to the heart itself.

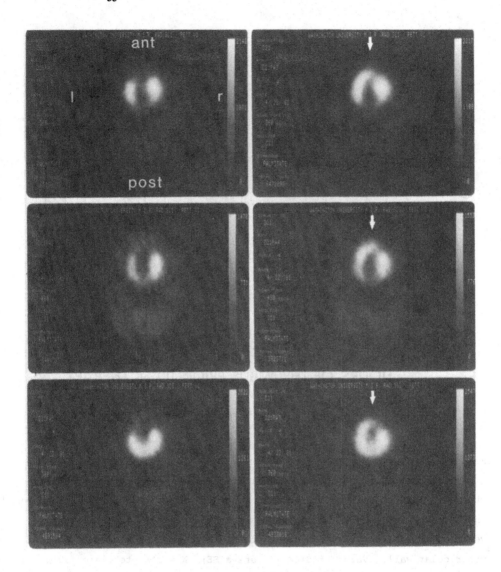

Figure 1

Three contiguous midventricular transverse positron emission tomograms obtained before (left) and after (right) thrombolysis. In this dog the initial tomogram was obtained 1.5 hours after occlusion following the intravenous administration of ^{11}C-palmitate. Intracoronary streptokinase was then given, and a second tomogram obtained one and a half hours after the first scan following a second injection of palmitate. With early reperfusion, the initial anterior defect fills in substantially on the second tomogram (arrow), indicating myocardial salvage (13). (Reprinted with permission from Technical Publishing Company).

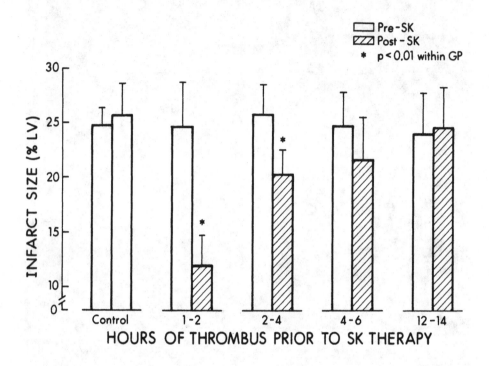

Figure 2

Histogram of tomographically estimated infarct size in all groups
studied. Infarct size refers to the extent of compromised zones defined based
on the number of pixels containing less than 50 percent of peak left
ventricular wall activity divided by the total number of pixels in the left
ventricular wall. Values indicate means ± SE; SK = streptokinase (13).
(Reprinted with permission from Technical Publishing Company).

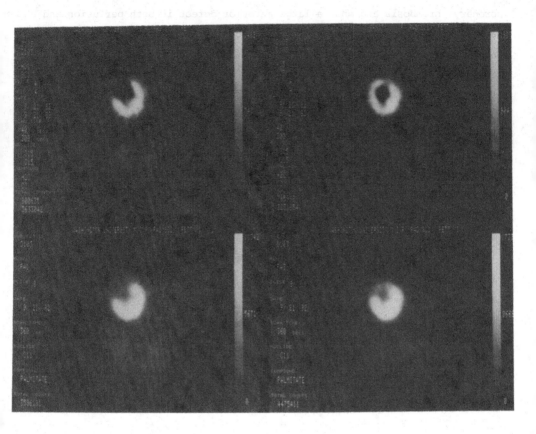

Figure 3

These reconstructions are from a single mid-ventricular transverse slice
obtained with PET before (top left and bottom left) and after (top right and
bottom right) thrombolysis in one dog treated with intravenous t-PA. In these
tomograms, anterior is to the top, posterior is to the bottom, and the free
lateral and septal walls of the left ventricle are to the reader's left and
right, respectively. The right ventricle is not visualized because of its
thin size. the top two panels show perfusion scans obtained after a bolus
injection of $H_2^{15}O$ with correction for vascular pool activity with
$C^{15}O$-labeled red blood cells before (left) and after (right) thrombolysis.
The bottom two panels show metabolism after the administration of
^{11}C-palmitate before (left) and after (right) thrombolysis. The
^{11}C-palmitate tomograms were corrected analogously for radioactivity in the
blood pool by using C^{15O}-labeled red blood cells to identify the vascular
space. The initial tomograms were obtained for 1 1/2 hours after induced

coronary thrombosis and show a large anterior defect in both perfusion and metabolism scans. The post-thrombolysis scans were obtained 1 1/2 hours after the first scan and approximately 80 minutes after thrombolysis following a second administration of $H_2^{15}O$, $C^{15}O$ and ^{11}C-palmitate. Restoration of perfusion is virtually complete. Significant restoration of ^{11}C-palmitate accumulation occurred, but a residual metabolic defect persisted in the center of the initially ischemic zone, consistent with death of some cells after ischemia of this duration. Total counts collected were greater than 800,000 in each scan, and the scale factor represents counts per pixel (16). (Reprinted with permission from the American Association for the Advancement of Science).

REFERENCES

1. Ishikawa, Y., George, S.E., Spaite, D., Hashimoto, H., Sobel, B.E., and
    Roberts, R.: Distortion of plasma CK curves induced by reperfusion:
    Mechanisms and implications. Circulation 68 (Suppl. III): III-196, 1983.

2. Wevers R.A., Wolters, R.J. and Soons, J.B.J.: Isoelectric focusing and
    hybridization experiments on creatine kinase (EC 2.7.3.2.). Clin. Chim.
    Acta 78:271, 1977.

3. Morelli, R., Carlson, C.J., Emilson, B., Abendschein, D.R. and Rapaport,
    E: Serum creatine kinase MM isoenzyme sub-bands after acute myocardial
    infarction in man. Circulation 67:1283, 1983.

4. Hashimoto, H., Grace, A.M., Billadello, J.J., Gross, R.W., Strauss, A.W.
    and Sobel, B.E.: Non-denaturing quantification of subforms of canine MM
    creatine kinase isoenzymes (isoforms) and their interconversion. J. Lab.
    Clin. Med., in press.

5. Sobel, B.E. and Bergmann, S.R.: Coronary thrombolysis: Some unresolved
    issues. Am. J. Med. 72:1, 1982.

6. Roberts, R., Sobel, B.E., and Ludbrook, P.A.: Determination of the
    origin of elevated plasma CPK after cardiac catherization. Cathet.
    Cardiovasc. Diagn. 2:329, 1976.

7. Weiss, E.S., Ahmed, S.A., Welch, M.J., Williamson, J.F., Ter-Pogossian,
    M.M. and Sobel, B.E.: Quantification of infarction in cross sections of
    canine myocardium in vivo with positron emission transaxial tomography
    and ^{11}C-palmitate. Circulation 55:66, 1977.

8. Sobel, B.E., Weiss, E.S., Welch, M.J., Siegel, B.A., and Ter-Pogossian,
    M.M.: Detection of remote myocardial infarction in patients with
    positron emission transaxial tomography and intravenous ^{11}C-palmitate.
    Circulation 55:853, 1977.

9. Ter-Pogossian, M.M., Klein, M.S., Markham, J., Roberts, R., and Sobel,
    B.E.: Regional assessment of myocardial metabolic integrity in vivo by
    positron-emission tomography with ^{11}C-labeled palmitate. Circulation
    61:242, 1980.

10. Sobel, B.E. and Geltman, E.M.: Localization and quantification of
    myocardial ischemia and infarction with postron emission tomography. In:
    Cardiovascular Medicine, Volume 1. Edited by John H.K. Vogel, New York,
    Raven Press, 1982.

11. Fox, K.A.A., Nomura, H., Sobel, B.E. and Bergmann, S.R.: Consistent substrate utilization despite reduced flow in hearts with maintained work. Am. J. Physiol. 13:H799, 1983.

12. Bergmann, S.R., Fox, K.A.A., Rand, A.L., Markham, J. and Sobel, B.E.: Quantitation of myocardial perfusion with radiolabeled water. J. Am. Coll. Cardiol. 1:577, 1983.

13. Bergmann, S.R., Lerch, R.A., Fox, K.A.A., Ludbrook, P.A., Welch, M.J., Ter-Pogossian M.M., and Sobel, B.E.: Temporal dependence of beneficial effects of coronary thrombolysis characterized by positron tomography. Am. J. Med. 73:573, 1982.

14. Ludbrook, P.A., Geltman, E.M., Tiefenbrunn, A.J., Jaffe, A.S., and Sobel, B.E.: Restoration of regional myocardial metabolism by coronary thrombolysis in patients. Circulation 68 (Suppl. III): -III-325, 1983.

15. Collen, D. and Verstraete, M.: Systemic thrombolytic therapy of acute myocardial infarction. Circulation 68:462, 1983.

16. Bergmann, S.R., Fox, K.A.A., Ter-Pogossian, M.M., and Sobel, B.E. (Washington University) and Collen, D. (University of Leuven): clot-selective coronary thrombolysis with tissue-type plasminogen activator. Science 220:1181, 1983.

6

MEASUREMENT OF MYOCARDIAL INFARCT SIZE USING NUCLEAR CARDIOLOGY METHODS

James T. Willerson, MD, Samuel E. Lewis, MD, James R. Corbett, MD,
Christopher L. Wolfe, MD, Robert W. Parkey, MD, and L. Maximilian Buja, MD

SUMMARY

The extent of myocardial infarction is an important predictor of patient course during the initial several months following acute myocardial infarction. Recently, several radionuclide methods have been developed that may provide insight into the extent of myocardial infarction. This review describes these methods, indicates their usefulness and limitations, and suggests a strategy for further development in the future.

INTRODUCTION

Infarct size is an important predictor of patient prognosis after acute myocardial infarction (1). Several Nuclear Cardiology procedures that utilize single photon emitters can provide information relative to infarct size in patients. Acute myocardial infarcts may be detected with the infarct-avid imaging agent, technetium-99m stannous pyrophosphate (Tc-99m-PPi) (2-5) and infarct size estimated from the extent of pyrophosphate uptake (6-8). Alternatively, acute myocardial infarcts may be detected as a perfusion defect on a thallium-201 myocardial scintigram and infarct size estimated from the extent of the perfusion defect (9-11). The functional impact of acute and chronic myocardial infarction on left and right ventricular performance can be estimated from radionuclide ventriculograms (12) and the extent of "jeopardized myocardium" predicted on the basis of rest and exercise radionuclide ventriculograms performed several weeks to months after the event (13,14). This review will focus on each of these three capabilities provided by Nuclear Cardiology methods, i.e. infarct detection and sizing with infarct-avid imaging, infarct detection and sizing with myocardial perfusion imaging, and the detection of the functional impact of acute and chronic myocardial infarction on ventricular performance and estimating the extent of jeopardized myocardium from rest and exercise radionuclide ventriculograms.

INFARCT DETECTION AND SIZING USING INFARCT-AVID
MYOCARDIAL SCINTIGRAPHY

Tc-99m-PPi is presently the agent of choice for the myocardial scinti-graphic detection and localization of acute myocardial infarction (2-5,15-21). Studies at our institution have demonstrated that it has approximately 90% sensitivity in infarct detection for acute myocardial infarcts equal to or greater than 3 grams in size when planar or two dimensional imaging is utilized (5-8,17,19-21). Tc-99m-PPi uptake occurs in irreversibly damaged myocardial cells almost exclusively (5,17,19) and its uptake is dependent upon there being a) some flow to the area of irreversible cellular damage, and b) calcium deposition within the severely injured myocardial cells (5,17,19). Clinicopathologic studies performed in patients have demonstrated that an abnormal Tc-99m-PPi myocardial scintigram usually identifies the presence of acute myocardial necrosis (5,17,19,21). Thus, this imaging technique provides a sensitive and relatively specific means to identify acute myocardial necrosis within the initial 24-96 hours after its occurrence.

1.   Procedural Details

Several technical details are important in obtaining high quality Tc-99m-PPi myocardial scintigrams. First, one injects 15-20 mCi Tc-99m coupled to 5 mg of stannous pyrophosphate intravenously and allows approximately 3 hours for the radionuclide blood pool to clear before obtaining myocardial scinti-grams in an anterior, shallow left anterior oblique (20°-30° left anterior oblique projection), a steep left anterior oblique projection (50°-60° left anterior oblique projection), and a left lateral projection. Ideally, at least 500,000 counts/projection are obtained. Second, some experience is required to distinguish increased Tc-99m-PPi uptake in bone, persistent radionuclide blood pool, and/or technically poor Tc-99m-PPi myocardial scintigrams from the presence of acute myocardial necrosis. Third, Tc-99m-PPi myocardial images should be obtained 24-96 hours after suspected myocardial infarction for maximal sensitivity in infarct detection (3-5). This time interval is optimal for Tc-99m-PPi imaging because this period is often required for a) important collateral flow to develop to the damaged myocardial region, and b) calcium deposition to develop within the area of infarction. Five days or more after myocardial infarction approximately fifty percent of the Tc-99m-PPi myocardial scintigrams become negative as the acute myocardial necrosis with calcium deposition is replaced by inflammatory debris and scar tissue

(5,17,19). However, if one uses Tc-99m-PPi myocardial scintigraphy in conjunction with lysing coronary thombi after acute myocardial infarction, the Tc-99m-PPi myocardial scintigram may become positive within 1-2 hours of the event (22). Precisely how soon Tc-99m-PPi myocardial scintigrams become negative with reperfusion is uncertain, but they may become negative sooner than occurs with permanent coronary arterial occlusion.

Planar or two dimensional myocardial imaging with Tc-99m-PPi myocardial scintigrams detects almost all myocardial infarcts equal to or larger than 3 grams in size within the time period of 24 hours to 5 days after the event. Sometimes, serial myocardial imaging is necessary to detect myocardial infarction especially when extensive coronary arterial stenoses and relatively poor reflow capability exist following acute myocardial infarction (23). However, tomographic imaging with single photon tomographic systems allows the detection of infarcts as small as one gram in experimental animal models (6-8,17) and we believe that it will allow the detection of relatively small infarcts in patients (24,25).

2. Sizing Acute Myocardial Infarcts with Infarct-Avid Imaging Agents

Acute transmural anterior or anterolateral infarcts may be sized accurately with planar imaging and area estimates of infarct size (Figure 2) (20). However, accurate sizing of inferior and nontransmural (subendocardial) myocardial infarcts requires three dimensional or tomographic imaging using single photon tomographic systems (SPECT) (6-8). We have shown that SPECT and imaging approaches that simulate three dimensional reconstruction of infarcts (26) allow the detection of myocardial infarcts as small as one gram and accurate estimation of infarct size independent of infarct location in animal models (8,26). Therefore, for accurate infarct sizing in patients, SPECT imaging with Tc-99m-PPi scintigraphy will be necessary.

3. Other Infarct-Avid Imaging Agents

Several other infarct-avid imaging agents have been described as useful in experimental animals and in preliminary studies in patients (27,28). In particular, a specific antibody to cardiac myosin has been shown to accumulate in irreversibly damaged myocardium and to allow infarct detection in experimental animals and in preliminary clinical evaluations (27). However, this antibody may have certain risks including a risk of anaphylaxis, if it should be necessary to use it serially for purposes of infarct detection or sizing in individual patients.

THALLIUM-201 MYOCARDIAL PERFUSION IMAGING

An alternative to infarct-avid imaging is the use of myocardial perfusion agents that accumulate in proportion to coronary blood flow in the myocardium and allow the detection of myocardial infarction as a void or defect in the myocardial perfusion scintigram (9-11). Thallium-201, a potassium analog, accumulates in the myocardium in proportion to coronary blood flow and does provide a means to detect acute myocardial infarction (and acute myocardial ischemia) by failing to accumulate in regions where coronary blood flow is significantly decreased (9-11,29-31). Thallium-201 has been used by Wackers, et al to detect acute myocardial infarction with a sensitivity of approximately 90% within the first 6-8 hours after myocardial infarction (9,10). However, if one delays obtaining a thallium-201 myocardial scintigram for more than 24 hours after suspected infarction, the sensitivity of the tests falls sharply. This is probably the result of increased collateral flow reaching the area of myocardial damage and reducing the extent of the perfusion defect, such that relatively small and moderate sized lesions may be missed by this imaging approach. It should also be emphasized that thallium-201 perfusion defects represent both myocardial necrosis and the extent of myocardial ischemia as they coexist after myocardial infarction rather than being a specific measure of new and/or old infarct size.

1. Procedural Details

Thallium-201 has a half life of approximately 72 hours and imaging should begin immediately after the intravenous injection of 1.5-2.0 mCi. If one waits even 10-15 minutes to begin imaging after the intravenous injection of thallium-201, some myocardial redistribution may occur causing one to miss small perfusion defects (32). Thallium-201 is relatively expensive and is ordinarily obtained from some distance so that imaging is made somewhat more difficult by these requirements. The same projections obtained for Tc-99m-PPi imaging are often used with Tl-201 imaging and interpretation of Tl-201 studies is made more accurate and objective by quantitative determination of Tl-201 uptake and washout (30) (Figure 3) and sensitivity and specificity will be enhanced further with the use of SPECT (33).

2. Sizing Acute Myocardial Infarcts

Silverman, et al have demonstrated that one may use the relative size of the thallium-201 perfusion defect to estimate infart size in patients and thus predict prognosis following the event (11). Those patients with the largest thallium-201 perfusion defects have the poorest prognosis in the several months following acute myocardial infarction (11).

RADIONUCLIDE VENTRICULOGRAPHY

Radionuclide ventriculography may be utilized to detect the functional impact of acute myocardial infarction on left and right ventricular performance (12). This is an important advantage since it is difficult to recognize the extent of ventricular damage in the patient with acute myocardial infarction at the bedside simply by using a stethoscope, chest x-ray, and detailed physical examination. It is well recognized that one may underestimate the severity of ventricular dysfunction without an objective measurement, such as can be provided with radionuclide ventriculography (Figure 4) (12). Sanford, et al at our institution have demonstrated a wide range of left ventricular ejection fractions obtained from radionuclide ventriculography in patients with varying Killip classification after acute myocardial infarction (12) (Figure 4). Specifically, patients in Killip I and II classifications may have either normal or severely depressed left ventricular ejection fractions; the knowledge of the relative severity of left ventricular functional abnormalities is helpful in a) selecting proper therapy for patients, b) determining the need for particularly careful observation of patients throughout their hospital stay, and c) developing the best diagnostic and therapeutic approaches for the future.

1.   Procedural Details

One may obtain radionuclide ventriculographic evaluation of ventricular function using either a) first pass or b) equilibrium studies and especially multigated image acquisition or "MUGA imaging" (34-36) (Figure 5). First pass imaging is obtained by injecting a radionuclide bolus into a central vein and following its passage through the right and into the left heart. Ordinarily, one uses technetium-99m pertechnetate or Tc-99m labeled red blood cells injected into a central vein and follows the passage of the radionuclide bolus. Accurate estimates of right ventricular function can be made if one "gates" the images that are acquired by subdividing the cardiac cycle into approximately 16 different segments, using the electrocardiogram coupled to the computer to identify various portions of the cardiac cycle and follows the 5-8 heart beats associated with entry of the radionuclide bolus into and through the right heart. Alternatively, one may use gated or equilibrium myocardial imaging where one identifies end-diastole and end-systole using the electrocardiogram or preferably obtains radionuclide counts from 16-32 segments of each cardiac cycle ("MUGA imaging") providing continuous information about cardiac systole and diastole. The MUGA studies may then be reviewed in a movie style foremat. We prefer the MUGA imaging approach and have used it to evaluate left and right ventricular function, including ejection fraction, ventricular volumes, and regional wall motion in patients within the initial 8 hours following acute myocardial infarction (12).

MUGA images are obtained after labeling the patient's red blood cells with Tc-99m pertechnetate (35). One has the half-life of Tc-99m pertechnetate, approximately 6 hours, to evaluate left and right ventricular function and an opportunity to establish the functional impact of any intervention that might be utilized on ventricular performance. The specific procedural details for obtaining gated images will not be described in detail here, but such information is available in many previous publications (12-14,35). Suffice it to say that one obtains images of the left and right ventricle in the anterior, modified left anterior oblique (30°-40° left anterior oblique with 5°-10° of caudal tilt of the imaging camera), 70° left anterior oblique, and left lateral views. At least 300,000 counts/image should be obtained and then with the help of an interactive computer, the ejection fraction may be calculated, regional wall motion estimated, and ventricular volumes measured accurately without geometric assumptions (35).

2. Sizing of Infarcts and Estimation of Extent of Jeopardized Myocardium

Measurement of left and right ventricular ejection fraction and of left ventricular volumes allows an accurate assessment of the extent of ventricular dysfunction caused by acute and chronic myocardial infarction (12). Initial measurements of ventricular function within hours of the infarct identifies the extent of irreversible damage and of superimposed myocardial ischemia as it affects ventricular performance. In the several days after the event, measurements of ventricular function provide a more exact estimate of the functional impact of the infarct on ventricular performance. Moreover, one may overlay the Tc-99m-PPi myocardial scintigram against the blood pool background allowing one to assign alterations in regional and global function to myocardial infarction and to identify areas of regional dysfunction outside the acute infarct zone (18). It is well recognized that patients after infarction with left ventricular ejection fractions at rest below 40 percent are at risk for future ischemic events, including sudden death (37).

At the time of hospital discharge one may utilize submaximal exercise testing with radionuclide ventriculography to identify patients at risk for future ischemic events (13,14) (Figure 6). Patients who demonstrate a decline in their left ventricular ejection fraction and an increase in left ventricular end-systolic volume with submaximal exercise at the time of hospital discharge are at risk for future ischemic events including new myocardial infarction and death (13,14). In contrast, those patients who have normal left ventricular functional responses to submaximal exercise at the time of hospital discharge have a good prognosis in the subsequent 6-8 months (13,14).

DISCUSSION

Nuclear cardiology methods may be utilized to detect and localize acute myocardial infarcts, estimate the extent of myocardial ischemia and of irreversible myocardial damage caused by myocardial infarction, assess the functional impact of acute and chronic myocardial infarction on ventricular performance, judge the efficacy of various interventions in altering ventricular function after myocardial infarction, and estimate prognosis in patients in the several months after the event. The methods that are utilized are relatively noninvasive, painless, essentially without risk to the patient except for the risk of low level radiation, and they may be repeated almost as often as necessary as long as one pays attention to the total radiation the patient receives.

It appears that single photon emission computed tomography will be an important addition and one that will provide quantitative information concerning infarct size, alterations in myocardial perfusion, and even the extent of regional wall motion abnormalities both at rest and during stress in patients that are studied (8,33,38). Planar or two dimensional imaging does not allow an accurate assessment of the overall extent of alterations in perfusion, regional ventricular function, or of infarct size located on the diaphragmatic surface of the heart and/or subendocardially. However, single photon emission tomographic systems are in their earliest stages of development and must improve further. Specifically, the instrumentation itself must improve such that resolution increases from centimeters to millimeters. The imaging systems must be made available at a reasonable expense. Moreoever, the necessary software to allow relatively rapid image reconstruction and display requires further development. It appears likely that such developments will occur during the next several years, thereby making available good alternatives to positron emission tomography for purposes of studying and detecting acute myocardial infarction, demonstrating alterations in myocardial perfusion, and evaluating global and segmental ventricular function.

Recent studies suggest that it may also be possible to use single photon emitters coupled to synthetic fatty acids to evaluate myocardial metabolism and perhaps estimate myocardial perfusion (39,40).

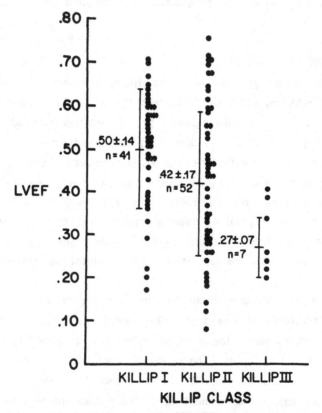

Figure 1: Panels A-C demonstrate a Tc-99m-PPi myocardial scintigram in a patient with an acute anterior myocardial infarction in the anterior (A), left anterior oblique (B), and left lateral (C) projections. The middle panels (D-F) demonstrate the same imaging projections and the usefulness of computer processing of the scintigrams to remove some of the bone background and provide an improved display of the abnormal region of pyrophosphate uptake. The bottom panels (G-I) demonstrate the site of an acute anterior myocardial infarction in the different imaging projections.

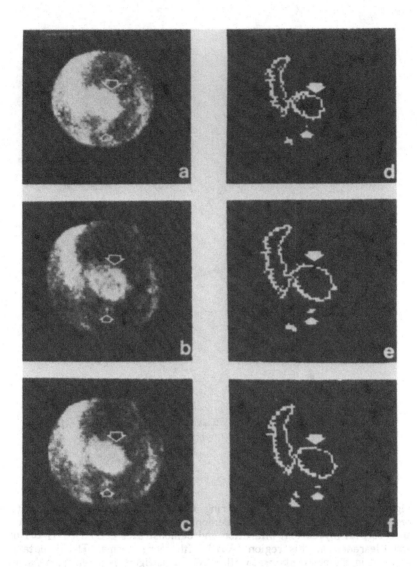

Figure 2: A large anterior myocardial infarction as identified by Tc-99m-PPi scintigraphy is shown in panels a-c and a computer-assisted method for identifying the area of increased pyrophosphate uptake is demonstrated in panels d-f.

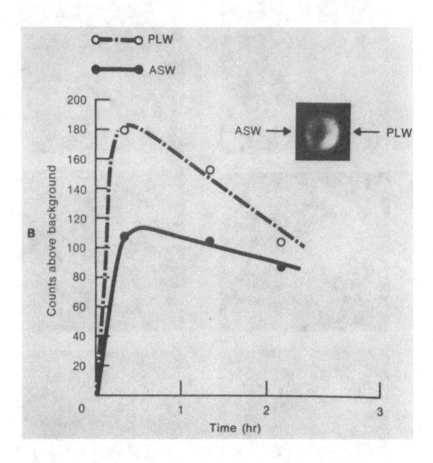

Figure 3. A technique for measuring Tl-201 uptake and washout in different regions of the left ventricle is demonstrated. This patient had a previous anteroseptal myocardial infarction and demonstrates decreased Tl-201 uptake and clearance in this region (ASW) with more normal Tl-201 uptake and washout in the posterolateral wall (PLW). This figure is taken from <u>Cardiovascular Nuclear Medicine</u>, page 233, editors H William Strauss and Bertram Pitt, C.V. Mosby Company, 1979 by permission.

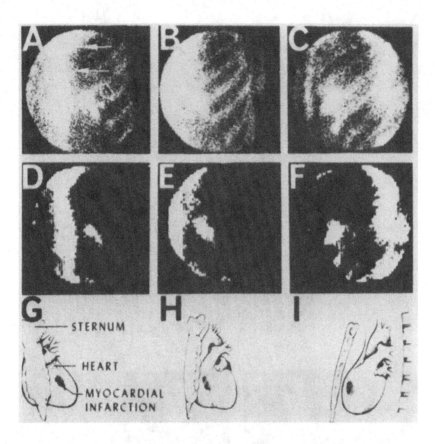

Figure 4. Correlations between left ventricular ejection fraction (vertical axis) and the Killip clinical classification of heart failure (horizontal axis) in patients with acute myocardial infarction studied within 8 hours of the event are shown. Note the wide spectrum of left ventricular ejection fractions in patients with no clinical evidence of heart failure (Killip I) and in those with moderate heart failure clinically (Killip II). This figure is taken from Am J Cardiology 49:637-644, 1982 with permission from the American Heart Association.

72

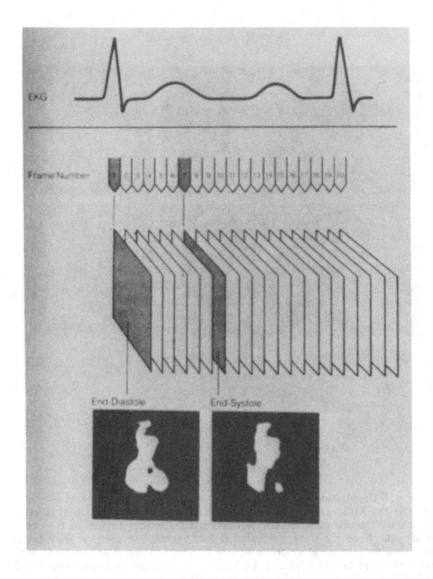

Figure 5. A schematic representation of multi-gated image acquisition analysis (MUGA imaging) is demonstrated. Radionuclide counts are summed from many different subsets of the cardiac cycle during systole and diastole and then may be played back in a movie style format for viewing as a continuous analysis of cardiac function.

REFERENCES

1. Page DL, Caulfield JB, Kastor JA, DeSanctis RW, Sanders CA: Myocardial changes associated with cardiogenic shock. N Engl J Med (285):133-137, 1971.
2. Bonte FJ, Parkey RW, Graham KD, Moore J, Stokely EM: A new method for radionuclide imaging of myocardial infarcts. Radiology (110):473-474, 1974.
3. Willerson JT, Parkey RW, Bonte FJ, Meyer SL, Atkins JM, Stokely EM: Technetium stannous pyrophosphate myocardial scintigrams in patients with chest pain of varying etiology. Circulation (51):1046-1052, 1975.
4. Parkey RW, Bonte FJ, Meyer SL, Atkins JM, Curry GC, Willerson JT: A new method for radionuclide imaging of myocardial infarction in humans. Circulation (50):540-546, 1974.
5. Buja LM, Parkey RW, Stokely EM, Bonte FJ, Willerson JT: Pathophysiology of technetium-99m stannous pyrophosphate and thallium-201 scintigraphy of canine acute myocardial infarcts. J Clin Invest (57):1508-1522, 1976.
6. Stokely EM, Tipton DM, Buja LM, Lewis SE, DeVous MD, Bonte FJ, Parkey RW, Willerson JT: Quantitation of experimental canine infarct size using multipinhole single photon tomography. J Nucl Med (22):55-61, 1981.
7. Lewis SE, Stokely EM, DeVous MD, Bonte FJ, Buja LM, Parkey RW, Willerson JT: Quantitation of experimental canine infarct size with multipinhole and rotating slanthole tomography. J Nucl Med 22:1000-1005, 1981.
8. Lewis SE, Devous MD Sr, Corbett JR, Izquierdo C, Nicod P, Wolfe CL, Parkey RW, Buja LM, Willerson JT: Measurement of infarct size in acute canine myocardial infarction by single photon emission computed tomography with technetium-99m pyrophosphate. Submitted.
9. Wackers FJ III, Schoot JB, Sokole EB, Niftrik GJ, Lie KI, Durrer D, Wellens HJJ: Noninvasive visualization of acute myocardial infarction in man with thallium-201. Brit Hrt J (37):741-744, 1975.
10. Wackers FJ, Sokole EB, Samson G, Schoot JB, Lie KI, Liem KL, Wellens HJJ: Value and limitations of thallium-201 scintigraphy in the acute phase of myocardial infarction. N Engl J Med (295):1-5, 1975.
11. Silverman KJ, Becker LC, Bulkley BH, Burow RD, Mellits ED, Kallman CH, Weisfeldt ML: Value of early thallium-201 scintigraphy for predicting mortality in patients with acute myocardial infarction. Circulation (61):996-1003, 1980.
12. Sanford CF, Corbett J, Curry GL, Lewis SE, Dehmer GJ, Anderson A, Moses B, Willerson JT: Value of radionuclide ventriculography in the immediate characterization of patients with acute myocardial infarction. Am J Cardiol (49):637-644, 1982.
13. Corbett J, Dehmer GJ, Lewis SE, Woodward W, Henderson E, Parkey RW, Blomqvist CG, Willerson JT: The prognostic value of submaximal exercise testing with radionuclide ventriculography prior to hospital discharge in patients with recent myocardial infarction. Circulation (64):535-544, 1981.
14. Corbett JR, Nicod P, Lewis SE, Rude RE, Willerson JT: Prognostic value of submaximal exercise radionuclide ventriculography following acute transmural and nontransmural myocardial infarction. Am J Cardiol (52):82A-91A, 1983.

15. Rude R, Parkey RW, Bonte FJ, Twieg D, Lewis S, Pulido J, Buja LM, Willerson JT: Clinical implications of the "doughnut" pattern of uptake in technetium-99m stannous pyrophosphate myocardial scintigrams in patients with acute myocardial infarction. Circulation (59):721-730, 1979.

16. Willerson JT, Parkey RW, Bonte F, Lewis S, Corbett J, Buja LM: Pathophysiologic considerations and clinicopathological correlates of technetium-99m stannous pyrophosphate myocardial scintigraphy. Semin Nucl Med (10):54-69, 1980.

17. Buja LM, Poliner L, Parkey RW, Pulido J, Hutcheson D, Platt MR, Mills L, Bonte FJ, Willerson JT: Clinicopathologic study of persistently positive technetium-99m stannous pyrophosphate myocardial scintigrams and myocytolytic degeneration after acute myocardial infarction. Circulation (56):1016-1023, 1977.

18. Corbett J, Lewis SE, Dehmer GJ, Bonte F, Parkey RW, Buja LM, Willerson JT: Simultaneous display of gated technetium-99m stannous pyrophosphate and dynamic LV myocardial scintigrams. J Nucl Med (22):671-677, 1981.

19. Buja LM, Tofe AJ, Kulkarni PV, Mukherjee A, Parkey RW, Francis MD, Bonte FJ, Willerson JT Sites and mechanisms of localization of technetium-99m phosphorus radiopharmaceuticals in acute myocardial infarcts and other tissues. J Clin Invest (60):724-740, 1977.

20. Willerson JT, Parkey RW, Stokely EM, Bonte FJ, Lewis SE, Harris RA Jr, Blomqvist CG, Poliner L, Buja LM: Infarct sizing with technetium-99m stannous pyrophosphate scintigraphy in dogs and man: relationship between scintigraphic and precordial mapping estimates of infarct size in patients. Cardiovas Res (11):291-299, 1977.

21. Poliner LR, Buja LM, Parkey RW, Bonte FJ, Willerson JT: Clinicopathologic findings in 52 patients studied by technetium-99m stannous pyrophosphate myocardial scintigraphy. Circulation (59):257-267, 1979.

22. Parkey RW, Kulkarni P, Lewis S, Datz F, Gutekunst D, Dehmer G, Buja L, Bonte F, Willerson JT: Effect of coronary blood flow and site of injection on Tc-99m-PPi detection of early canine myocardial infarcts. J Nucl Med (22):133-137, 1981.

23. Falkoff M, Parkey RW, Bonte FJ, Lewis S, Buja LM, Dehmer G, Willerson JT: Technetium-99m stannous pyrophosphate myocardial scintigraphy: The need for serial imaging to detect myocardial infarcts in patients. Clinical Cardiol (1):163-168, 1978.

24. Corbett JR, Lewis M, Willerson JT, Nicod PH, Huxley RL, Simon T, Henderson E, Parkey R, Rellas JS, Sokolov JJ, Lewis SE: Technetium-99m pyrophosphate imaging in acute myocardial infarction: Comparison of planar images with single-photon tomography with blood pool overlay. Submitted.

25. Corbett JR, Lewis SE, Wolfe CL, Rellas JS, Lewis M, Parkey RW, Sokolov JJ, Rude RE, Buja LM, Willerson JT: Measurement of myocardial infarct size in patients by technetium pyrophosphate single photon tomography. Submitted.

26. Lewis M, Buja LM, Saffer S, Mishelevich D, Stokely E, Lewis S, Parkey R, Bonte F, Willerson JT: Experimental infarct sizing utilizing computer processing and a three-dimensional model. Science (197):167-169, 1977.

27. Khaw BA, Beller GA, Haber E, et al: Localization and sizing of myocardial infarcts employing radioactivity labeled myosin specific antibody. Clin Res (23):381A, 1975 (abstr).

28. Holman BL, Lesch M, Zweiman FG, Temte J, Lown B, Gorlin R: Detection and sizing of acute myocardial infarcts with $^{99m}Tc(Sn)$ tetracycline. N Engl J Med (291):159-163, 1974.

29. Strauss HW, Harrison K, Langan JK, Lebowitz E, Pitt B: Thallium-201 for myocardial imaging: relation of thallium-201 to regional myocardial perfusion. Circulation (51):641-645, 1975.

30. Beller GA, Watson DD, Pohost GM: Kinetics of thallium distribution and redistribution: clinical application in segmental myocardial imaging. In Strauss HW, Pitt B (ed) Cardiovascular Nuclear Medicine. 2nd ed. Mosby Press, St. Louis, 1979, p 225.

31. Burrow RD, Pond M, Shafer AW, Becker L: Circumferential profiles: a new method for computer analysis of thallium-201 myocardial perfusion images. J Nucl Med (20):771-777, 1979.

32. Pohost GM, Zir LM, Moore RH, McKusick KA, Guiney TE, Beller GA: Differentiation of transiently ischemic from infarcted myocardium by serial imaging after a single dose of thallium-201. Circulation (55):294-302, 1977.

33. Ritchie JL, Williams DL, Harp G, Stratton JL, Caldwell JH: Transaxial tomography with thallium-201 for detecting remote myocardial infarction. Comparison with planar imaging. Am J Cardiol (50):1236-1241, 1982.

34. Berger HJ, Reduto LA, Johnstone DE, Borkowski H, Sands JM, Cohen LS, Langou RA, Gottschalk A, Zaret BL: Global and regional left ventricular response to bicycle exercise in coronary artery disease: assessment by quantitative radionuclide angiocardiography. Am J Med (66):13-21, 1979.

35. Dehmer GJ, Lewis SE, Hillis LD, Corbett J, Parkey RW, Willerson JT: Exercise induced alterations in left ventricular volumes in man: usefulness in predicting the relative extent of coronary artery disease. Circulation (63):1008-1018, 1981.

36. Borer JS, Kent KM, Bacharach SL, Green MV, Rosing DR, Seides SF, Epstein SE, Johnston GS: Sensitivity, specificity and predictive accuracy of radionuclide cineangiography during exercise in patients with coronary artery disease. Circulation (60):572-580, 1979.

37. Mukharji J, Rude R, Gustafson N, Poole K, Passamani ER, Thomas LJ Jr, Strauss HW, Muller JE, Roberts R, Raabe DS, Braunwald E, Willerson JT, Cooperating Investigators, Multicenter Investigation of the Limitation of Infarct Size: Late sudden death following myocardial infarction: Interdependence of risk factors. J Am Coll Cardiol (1):585, 1983. (abstr)

38. Corbett J, Lewis S, Wolfe C, Rellas J, Lewis M, Parkey R, Sokolov J, Rude R, Buja LM, Willerson J: Measurement of myocardial infarct size by technetium pyrophosphate single photon tomography. Circulation (68):III-394, 1983.

39. Rellas JS, Corbett JR, Kulkarni P, Morgan C, Devous MD, Buja LM, Buja L, Parkey RW, Willerson JT, Lewis SE: Iodine-123 phenylpentadecanoic acid: Detection of acute myocardial infarction and injury using an iodinated fatty acid and single photon emission tomography. Am J Cardio (in press, 1983).

40. Rellas JS, Corbett JR, Kulkarni P, Morgan C, Devous M, Buja LM, Parkey RW, Willerson JT, Lewis SE: Iodine-123 phenylpentadecanoic acid: Detection of acute myocardial infarction in anesthetized dogs. In, Advances in Myocardiology. Plenum Publishing Co., New York, in press, 1983.

7

ECHOCARDIOGRAPHIC APPROACHES TO THE EVALUATION OF ACUTE MYOCARDIAL INFARCTION
I: Observations in Experimental Animals

Andrew J. Kemper, M.D.
Alfred F. Parisi, M.D.

Acute myocardial infarction is a dynamic process. Occlusion of a
coronary artery results in regional myocardial hypoperfusion. When
regional blood flow falls below the level needed to meet myocardial
demands active contraction is replaced by aneurysmal bulging in the
malperfused area (1). After 30-45 minutes of ischemia, a "wave" of
necrosis begins in the endocardium which progresses radially towards the
epicardium (2). After six hours necrosis is complete and healing begins
(2). Tissue edema swells the region of necrosis while inflammatory and
scavenger cells flood the area over the ensuing week (3). Collagenous
("scar") tissue is then deposited and the injured region shrinks in
size over the next six weeks (4,5).

Two-dimensional echocardiography is a method well suited to the
study of this dynamic process. High resolution real time images of
myocardial function and structure can be obtained repeatedly in the
experimental laboratory and in the clinical setting. Observations made
during coronary occlusion in experimental animals have led to three
major echocardiographic approaches to the quantification of acute
myocardial ischemia and infarction: 1) analysis of contractile
function; 2) direct imaging of myocardial perfusion using
echocardiographic contrast enhancing agents; and 3) signal processing of
reflected ultrasound as an index of underlying tissue changes. Each
approach will be considered in turn in this review.

Functional Analysis

In the five decades since Tennant and Wiggers first used epicardial
myographs to describe aneurysmal bulging of myocardium served by an acutely
ligated coronary artery (1), numerous studies have confirmed and

extended their observations. Regional contraction abnormalities were observed to occur within the myocardium itself rather than on its surface by Heyndrickx et al, using pairs of ultrasonic sonomicrometers implanted in the subendocardium (6). Gallagher et al, using paired sonomicrometers in an animal model with graded coronary occlusion, observed that decreased circumferential shortening and transmural thickening paralleled the degree of endocardial ischemia while the epicardial third of the myocardium was constrained from shortening, or "tethered", even in the presence of normal or increased epicardial flow (7). During transmural ischemia, circumferential lengthening and myocardial thinning were observed (7). These observations are similar to those made using conventional M-mode echocardiography by direct application of the transducer to the ventricular wall: 1) thinning and aneurysmal bulging in the central zone; 2) impaired thickening and decreased motion in marginal zones; 3) transitional abnormalities in adjacent zones; and 4) compensatory hyperactivity in healthy remote areas (8,9).

The first quantitative two-dimensional study performed in animals, by Meltzer et al (10), compared an index of infarction derived from segmental endocardial motion five hours following left anterior descending coronary artery occlusion with infarct size derived from pyrophosphate scanning. Although a correlation coefficient of 0.75 between these two measures was seen in 14 animals having infarction segmental motion underestimated infarct size significantly, perhaps because the single long axis view employed may not have adequately surveyed all areas of dysfunction.

Lieberman et al compared radial endocardial motion and systolic thickening 48 hours after occlusion as an indicator of morphologic myocardial infarction (11). Data was obtained in an open-chested model by use of a mechanical grid and transducer standoff device applied directly to the epicardial surface. In their study, although both abnormal endocardial excursion and failure to thicken occured in regions of infarction, thickening analysis was more accurate than endocardial motion analysis in distinguishing infarcted and non-infarcted tissue. More importantly, they observed that neither method reflected the transmural extent of infarction. Rather, a threshhold phenomenon was seen. All regions having greater than 20% transmural

FIGURE 1. Relationship between percentage of echocardiographic systolic wall thickening and transmural extent of infarct thickness measured histologically plotted in 20% increments. Regions having greater than 20% transmural infarction fail to thicken.(Reprinted with permission from Lieberman et al [11], courtesy of American Heart Association.)

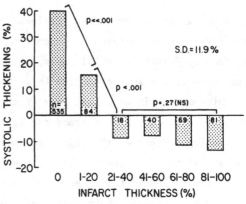

infarction failed to thicken. (Figure 1.) They suggested that this phenomenon might preclude accurate infarct size measurement for any method relying on functional analysis

Thickening analysis has the advantage of assessing transmural thickening and thinning as an intrinsic feature of myocardial contractile function which is independent of the swinging motion of the heart. This swinging motion confounds analysis of endocardial motion. However, analysis of endocardial thickening requires accurate definition of the relative motion of endocardial and epicardial targets which are usually separated by 10-15 millimeters. Since the lateral resolution of two-dimensional echocardiographic systems is in the range of 3-5 millimeters and becomes poorer at increasing tissue depths, the theoretical advantages of thickening analysis demonstrated in an open chested model may not be as useful in the clinical situation. O'Boyle et al, compared an area shrinkage method based on endocardial motion with wall thickening as indicators of myocardial infarction in a closed-chested canine model (12). No advantage was be demonstrated for either method (wall motion vs infarct extent: r=0.76, SEE=.16; thickening vs infarct extent: r=0.77, SEE=.16. Figure 2.) They concluded that both methods of analysis are equally effective in detecting and quantifying the extent of infarction.

The controversy regarding the proper method of quantifying regional left ventricular function as an indicator of myocardial infarction may be overshadowed by temporal changes which have been demonstrated to occur in the relationship between function and necrosis. Nieminen et al compared the fraction of the left ventricle which showed abnormal thickening at two, twenty-four and forty-eight hours after coronary ligation to the

FIGURE 2. A) Frequency distribution of the mean circumferential
extent of infarctions at pathologic examination not detected by two-
dimensional echocardiographic wall
thickening and endocardial motion
determined by area shrinkage
algorithm. B) Frequency of mean
circumferential extent of infarctions detected by each echocardiographic approach. (Reprinted courtesy of Technical Publishing Co.
[12]).

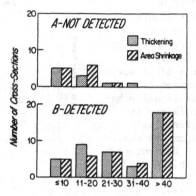

Mean Circumferential Extent of Infarction
at Pathology (%)

left ventricular fraction shown to be infarcted by pathologic
evaluation (13). Data were derived from a weighted summation of
abnormally contracting segments observed at three echocardiographic
cross-sectional levels in a closed-chested model. At two hours
following occlusion, the fraction of the ventricle showing abnormal
thickening markedly overestimated and correlated poorly with the
fraction shown to be necrosed. (25.3% abnormal function vs. 13.4%
infarcted; r=0.60). Infarct size predicted by thickening analysis
decreased over 48 hours but still correlated relatively poorly (15.3%
abnormal by thickening; r=0.73). (Figure 3.) These findings are
compatible with those of Ellis et al, who described a similar change in
the circumferential extent of abnormal thinning seen in mid-papillary
muscle level slices following acute occlusion (14). The percent of the
circumference which thinned decreased from 32% at ninety minutes to 11%
by 14 days following permanent occlusion.

During reperfusion of previously ischemic myocardium an even more
striking dissociation is seen between myocardial function and tissue
viability. Wyatt et al, found no correlation between the extent of
abnormal endocardial motion 48 hours after occlusion and infarct size in
short axis sections examined in six dogs that underwent three hours of
occlusion followed by reperfusion (15). In a similar experiment, Ellis
et al, observed the time course of functional recovery in animals
undergoing two hours of occlusion followed by reperfusion (14). Central
regions in the ischemic area which showed myocardial salvage failed to

FIGURE 3.
Relationship
of infarct size
determined patho-
logically 48
hours after occlu-
sion and two-
dimensional echo-
cardiographic
regional wall
motion abnormali-
ties determined
by thickening

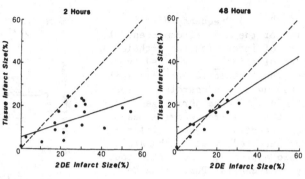

analysis (2DE) at two hours (left) and at 48 hours (right). The
regression equation (solid line) at two hours is y = 0.32x + 5.31%
(r=0.60, SEE=5.9%). The regression equation at 49 hours is y = 0.60x +
6.53% (r=0.73, SEE=4.9%). (Reprinted courtesy of American Heart
Association [13]).

show evidence of thickening until 72 hours following reperfusion.
These areas thickened to 39% of the pre-occlusion level by 14 days.
Peripheral ischemic areas showed some thickening by six hours and
nearly complete recovery by 14 days. No comment was made regarding
salvage or the transmural extent of infarction in this study (14).
These findings are similar to those recently observed in our laboratory
in a study designed to assess the reliability of wall motion analysis
as an indicator of the extent of myocardium salvaged by reperfusion
after hours of coronary occlusion (16). No significant improvement was
seen in regional ventricular function four hours following
reperfusion despite salvage of 60% of the myocardium within the
ischemic area.

Functional analysis relies on myocardial contractility as an index
of viability. Although thickening analysis is potentially more precise
than endocardial motion analysis in estimating infarct size,
difficulties in target recognition and the intrinsic dissociation
between contractile function and tissue integrity during acute ischemia
may obviate any advantages of thickening analysis. Most studies
indicate that functional analyses overestimate infarct size,
particularly during the critical early hours following occlusion.
Future modifications utilizing detailed temporal analysis of entire
cardiac cycles rather than comparison of single end diastolic and end
systolic frames may improve the accuracy of functional analysis.

However, at present, while this approach is of value in tracking the course of acute infarction, accurate assessment of the extent of left ventricular myocardium undergoing necrosis cannot be made using this technique.

Perfusion Imaging

Early studies using M—mode echocardiography demonstrated that an increase in intraventricular echocardiographic contrast could be achieved by the injection of solutions such as agitated saline and indocyanine green, which contain dissolved microbubbles. Bommer et al, demonstrated that left atrial or supra—aortic injection of specially prepared echo-reflective "microballoons"resulted in increased contrast in normally perfused myocardium (17). Armstrong et al, performed mid-papillary two-dimensional cross-sectional echocardiograms during supra-aortic injections of a specially prepared gelatin encapsulated microsphere solution in an open-chested canine model of acute coronary occlusion. Contrast enhancement, measured by a commercial light meter correctly identified 48/51 octants as having more or less than 50% normal flow as measured by the radioactive microsphere technique (18). More recently, interest has centered on two new methods which produce such an intense increase in myocardial contrast that in vivo real time imaging of regional perfusion is possible. They are intracoronary injection of an agitated renografin/saline mixture and supra-aortic injection of a dilute hydrogen peroxide and blood solution.

Tei et al showed good contrast enhancement could be obtained in myocardium perfused by vessels injected with a mixture of agitated saline and renograffin (19). This group has also presented preliminary data which shows that a good correlation exists between malperfusion shown by monstral blue staining and areas which fail to enhance during left main coronary artery injection in single slices obtained during coronary occlusion in an open-chested dog model (20).

Work recently done by Armstrong et al (21), and in our laboratory (22) has utilized the echocardiographic contrast enhancement engendered by supra-aortic injection of a dilute hydrogen peroxide and blood solution as a maker for myocardial perfusion. This method results in intense

82

FIGURE 4. Normal hy-
drogen peroxide echocar-
diographic study at the
high papillary level.
Baseline study (left)
shows clear endocardial
and epicardial target
definition with few
intramyocardial echoes.
Following peroxide injec-
tion (right), normal myo-
cardium is homogeneously
enhanced. Orientation
on left panel (S= septum,
A=anterior, L=lateral, P=posterior.)

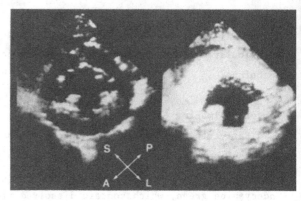

echocardiographic enhancement of normally perfused myocardium (Figure 4).
Contrast defects are clearly delineated (Figure 5). Armstrong et al,
showed a close correlation between contrast defects four hours after
occlusion and myocardial infarct size in single mid-papillary slices obtained in an open-chested model (r=0.92, SEE=0.05)(21). In our study using
a closed-chested model, a close correlation was seen between both
malperfusion, measured by monastral blue pigment, and infarction, measured
by TTC staining, and the extent of a contrast defect observed after six
hours of occlusion at four echocardiographic levels (r=0.93, SEE=7.7% vs.
malperfusion; r=0.89, SEE=8.9% vs. infarction) (22). In both studies (21,
22), contrast defect assessment was clearly superior to functional analysis
for the estimation of infarct size and region of malperfusion.

In a recently completed series of experiments, we investigated the
potential usefulness of hydrogen peroxide perfusion imaging in assessing
the extent of myocardium at risk during occlusion and the fraction of
myocardium at risk which was salvaged by reperfusion after 1 - 2 1/2 hours
of occlusion in 20 animals (23). The fraction of the ventricle involved
was calculated as a weighted sum of contrast defects observed at four
levels. The fraction of the ventricle which failed to enhance during
occlusion correlated well with the fraction of LV mass at risk using the
radioactive microsphere technique (r=0.89, SEE=4.5%). Three hours after
reperfusion, the fraction which showed abnormal perfusion by contrast
enhancement correlated well with the fraction of LV mass infarcted (r=0.84,
SEE=5.3%). The ratio of the echocardiographic contrast measures of risk

FIGURE 5. Representative contrast echocardiographic study at the high papillary level from an animal undergoing 120 minutes occlusion followed by reperfusion. During occlusion (left panel) contrast echocardiography disclosed a sharply bordered region of decreased contrast extending from 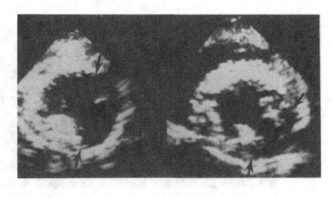 the posterior to the lateral wall (between arrows). During reperfusion (right panel), the contrast negative region (between arrows) is smaller and more regularly defined. The contrast negative region during perfusion correlated well with malperfusion shown by autoradiography and the contrast negative region during reperfusion correlated well with infarction shown by TTC staining.

and infarction had a significant correlation with morphologic measures of myocardium at risk which was salvaged by reperfusion (r=0.77, SEE=16.9%). Contrast echocardiograph correctly classified 18 of 20 animals as having more or less than 70% salvage of ischemic myocardium.

Echocardiographic contrast enhancement using supra-aortic hydrogen peroxide injection delineates myocardial perfusion. It is superior to wall motion analysis for the assessment of the ventricular fraction at risk during coronary occlusion. When contrast studies are performed during reperfusion, areas which enhance can be shown to be viable by morphologic techniques. The technique is simple to perform and readily repeatable. If hydrogen peroxide or a similar contrast enhancing agent can be shown to be safe, this approach may prove to have widespread applicability to the clinical problem of infarct assessment.

Echo Signal Processing

The course of healing of myocardial infarction at the cellular level is well described. An early phase of inflammation and edema is followed by neovascularization and fibroblastic activity which lead to collagen formation and scar contraction (4,5). These changes at the cellular level are accompanied by alterations in acoustic reflectivity which have been observed in M-mode studies as "increased echo density" in regions of myocardial scarring (24). Early in vitro "backscatter" experiments

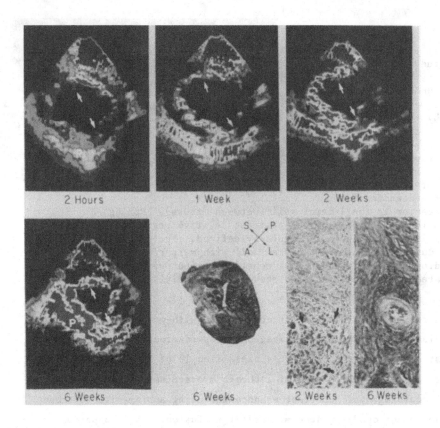

FIGURE 6. Serial two-dimensional echocardiograms from one dog
undergoing left anterior descending ligation with a gross pathologic
cross-section and microscopic histologic specimens from the level of
the infarctions. Myocardium to the left of the white arrows was akinetic
in real time observations. Two hours following ligation echo intensity
and distribution had not changed from baseline. From one to six weeks
following ligation there was a progressive increase in echo intensity
in the infarcted area, which when color-coded, changed from yellow at
one week to bright red by six weeks. Here reproduced in half-tone
black and white, these changes can be observed as a progressive increase
in shading in the infarcted areas. Similar changes in echo intensity
occurred in the pericardium (P) and are related to an adhesive pericardial
reaction. The gross pathologic cross-section in the same heart shows
an area of infarction which corresponds well with the shaded area in
the six-week echocardiogram. Intersecting arrows indicate orientation
of echocardiograms and gross section. S=septal; p=posterior;
L=lateral; A=Anterior. At bottom right are histologic sections.

demonstrated that increases in the frequency and amplitude of ultrasound

reflected from infarcted myocardium closely parallels increases in

collagen content (25,26). More recently, Mimbs et al, have demonstrated in vivo, using an open-chested canine model, similar but less intense changes in the characteristics of ultrasound reflected fromacutely ischemic areas (27).

Logan-Sinclair et al, demonstrated the potential application of amplitude processing to two-dimensional echocardiography (28). By color-coding signal amplitude, they were able to demonstrate that a consistent increase in intensity occurs in echoes reflected from abnormally fibrous tissue such as rheumatic valves or regions of left ventricular scar.

In a recent experimental study in our laboratory, the evolutionary changes accompanying the healing of acute myocardial infarction were studied using a similar color-encoded two-dimensional method (29). Echo intensity was seen to increase progressively over the course of six to eight weeks. The amplitude of reflected ultrasound increased two to three-fold and most closely paralleled the four-fold increase seen in collagen content in the infarcted area. At present this approach has important limitations because of the subject to subject variability that can occur in echo intensity due to the angle of dependence of reflected signal amplitude, specular reflections and gain dependency. However, it may prove to be of value in serial clinical studies during the course of infarction where the myocardium of each patient can be observed in reference to its findings on initial examination under circumstances where the transducer application and gain settings can be kept constant. The state of non-functioning myocardium might be quite different in two patients with acute infarction, one of whom develops diffuse high intensity echoes within the akinetic segment while the other does not. A great deal of further work needs to be done to define the relationships between echo characteristics and changes in tissue before this method can be used to quantify the extent of acute infarction.

This review has described three major echocardiographic approaches to the in vivo quantification of acute myocardial ischemia and infarction. At present only one of these, analysis of regional myocardial function, is applicable in the clinical situation. Further work using experimental animal models should focus on methods of improving functional analysis as a measure of risk area and infarction, developing contrast agents safe for use in the clinical situation, and further characterizing the nature of the relationship between reflected ultrasound and changes in tissue.

REFERENCES

1.   Tennant R, Wiggers CJ: The effect of coronary occlusion on myocardial contraction. Am J Physiol 112:351, 1935.
2.   Reimer KA, Jennings RB: The "wave front phenomenon" of myocardial cell death. Transmural progression of necrosis within the framework of ischemic bed size (myocardium at risk) and collateral flow. Laboratory Investigation 40:633, 1979.
3.   Reimer KA, Jennings RB: The changing anatomic reference base of evolving myocardial infarction. Circulation 60:866, 1979.
4.   Mallory GK, White PD, Salcedo-Salgar J: The speed of healing of myocardial infarction. A study of pathologic anatomy in seventy-two cases. Am Heart J 18:647, 1939.
5.   Fishbein MC, Maclean D, Maroko PR: The histologic evolution of myocardial infarction. Chest 73:843, 1978.
6.   Heyndrickx G, Millard RW, McRitchie RJ, Maroko PR, Vatner SF: Regional myocardial alterations after brief coronary artery occlusion in conscious dogs. J Clin Invest 56:987, 1975.
7.   Ghallagher KP, Osakada G, Hess OM, Koziol JA, Kemper WS, Ross JR, Jr.: Subepicardial segmental function during coronary stenosis and the role of myocardial fiber orientation. Circulation Research 50:352, 1982.
8.   Kerber RE, Abboud FM: Echocardiographic detection of regional myocardial infarction: an experimental study. Circulation 47:997-1005, 1973.
9.   Kerber RE, Marcus ML, Wilson R, Erhardt J, Abboud FM: Effects of acute coronary occlusion on the motion and perfusion of the normal and ischemic interventricular septum: an experimental echocardiographic study. Circulation 54:928-35, 1976.
10.   Meltzer RS, Woythaler JN, Buda AJ, et al: Two-dimensional echocardiographic quantification of infarct size alteration by pharmacologic agents. Am J Cardiol 44:257-62, 1979.
11.   Lieberman AN, Weiss JL, Jugdutt BI, Becker LC, Bulkley BH, Garrison JG, Hutchins GM, Kallman CA, Weisfeldt ML: Two-dimensional echocardiography and infarct size: relationship of regional wall motion and thickening to the extent of myocardial infarction in the dog. Circulation 63(4):739-46, 1981.
12.   O'Boyle JE, Parisi AF, Nieminen M, Kloner RA, Khuri S: Quantitative detection of regional left ventricular contraction abnormalities by two-dimensional echocardiography: comparison of myocardial thickening and thinning and endocardial motion in a canine model. Am J Cardiol 51:1732-38, 1983.
13.   Nieminen M, Parisi AF, O'Boyle JE, Folland ED, Khuri S, Kloner RA: Serial evaluation of myocardial thickening and thinning in acute experimental infarction: identification and quantification using two-dimensional echocardiograpy. Circulation 66(1):174-180, 1982.
14.   Elis SG, Henschke CI, Sandor T, Wynne J, Braunwald E, Kloner RA: Time course of functional and biochemical recovery of myocardium salvaged by reperfusion. J Am Coll Cardiol 1(4):1047-55, 1983.
15.   Wyatt HL, Meerbaum S, Heng MK, Rit J, Gueret P, Corday E: Experimental evaluation of the extent of myocardial dyssynergy and infarct size by two-dimensional echocardiography. Circulation 63(4):607-614, 1981.
16.   Hammerman H, O'Boyle JE, Cohen CA, Kloner RA, Parisi AF: Dissociation between two-dimensional echo wall motion and tissue salvage in early experimental myocardial infarction. (Submitted for publication.)

17. Bommer WJ, Rasor J, Tickner G, Takeda P, Miller L, Lee G, Mason DT, DeMaria AN: Quantitative regional myocardial perfusion scanning with contrast echocardiography. (Abstr.) Am J Cardiol 47:403, 1981.

18. Armstrong WF, Mueller TM, Kinney EL, Tickner EG, Dillon JC, Feigenbaum H: Assessment of myocardial perfusion abnormalities with contrast-enhanced two-dimensional echocardiography. Circulation 66:166, 1982.

19. Tei C, Sakamaki T, Shah PM, Meerbaum S, Shimoura K, Kondo S, Corday E: Myocardial contrast echocardiography: a reproducible technique of myocardial opacification for identifying regional perfusion deficits. Circulation 67:585, 1983.

20. Sakamaki T, Tei C, Meerbaum S, Kondo S, Shimoura K, Fishbein MC, Y-Rit J, Shah PM, Corday E: Validation of contrast two-dimensional echocardiography delineation of underperfused myocardium during acute ischemia. (Abstr.) Circulation 66:II-7, 1982.

21. Armstrong WF, West SR, Mueller TM, Dillon JC, Feigenbaum H: Assessment of location and size of myocardial infarction with contrast-enhanced echocardiography. J Amer Coll Cardiol 2:63, 1983.

22. Kemper AJ, O'Boyle JE, Sharma S, Cohen CA, Kloner RA, Khuri SF, Parisi AF: Hydrogen peroxide contrast-enhanced two-dimensional echocardiography: real-time in vivo delineation of regional myocardial perfusion. Circulation 68(3):603-611, 1983.

23. Kemper AJ, O'Boyle JE, Taylor A, Cohen CA, Khuri SF, Parisi AF: Supra-aortic hydrogen peroxide contrast echocardiography (SHPCE) during coronary occlusion: in vivo determination of myocardium at risk and extent of infarction following reperfusion. (Abstr.) Circulation 68 Suppl III, III-93, 1983.

24. Rasmussen S, Corya BC, Feigenbaum H, Knoebel SB: Detection of myocardial scar tissue by M-mode echocardiography. Circulation 57:230, 1978.

25. Gramiak R, Waag RC, Schenk EA, Lee PK, Thomson K, MacIntosh P: Ultrasonic detection of myocardial infarction by amplitude analysis. Radiology 130:713, 1979.

26. Mimbs JW, O'Donnell M, Bauwens D, Miller JW, Sobel BE: The dependence of ultrasonic attenuation and backscatter on collagen content in dog and rabbit hearts. Circ Res 47:49, 1980.

27. Mimbs JW, Bauwens D, Cohen RD, O'Donnell M, Miller JG, Sobel BE: Effects of myocardial ischemia on quantitative ultrasonic backscatter and identification of responsible determinants. Circ Res 49:89, 1981.

28. Logan-Sinclair R, Wong CM, Gibson DG: Clinical application of amplitude processing of echocardiographic images. Brit Heart J 45:621, 1981.

29. Parisi AF, Nieminen M, O'Boyle JE, Moynihan PF, Khuri SF, Kloner RA, Folland ED, Schoen FJ. Enhanced detection of the evolution of tissue changes after acute myocardial infarction using color-enhanced two-dimensional echocardiography. Circulation 66:764, 1982.

8

TWO DIMENSIONAL ECHOCARDIOGRAPHY IN ACUTE MYOCARDIAL INFARCTION:
CLINICAL APPLICATIONS

Ioannis P. Panidis, M.D. and Joel Morganroth, M.D.

INTRODUCTION:

The usefulness of echocardiography in the setting of acute
myocardial infarction has been extensively studied over the past
few years.   Early clinical studies demonstrated localized areas
of left ventricular asynergy in patients with acute myocardial
infarction (MI) utilizing M-mode echocardiography.   Two-
dimensional echocardiography with its superior spatial
orientation and display of the various left ventricular segments
in several views, allows reliable determination of the presence,
location and extent of wall motion abnormalities in acute MI.
Furthermore two dimensional echocardiography (2D-echo) can be
useful in detecting complications of acute MI and has potential
applications in screening patients with the chest pain syndrome
and determining the prognosis in patients with established MI.
(Table 1)

DIAGNOSIS OF ACUTE MI:

The presence of regional left ventricular wall motion
abnormality (hypokinesis, akinesis or dyskinesis) on 2D-echo

serves as a marker for coronary artery disease and usually represents an area of infarcted myocardium. Heger et al[1] found such abnormalities in each patient with clinically documented acute transmural MI studied by 2D-echo within 48 hours of admission. In this study the location of echocardiographic left ventricular asynergy correlated very well with the electrocardiographic location (Q-waves) of acute infarction.

In a study of 80 patients with acute chest pain admitted to an intensive care unit, regional wall motion abnormalities were identified by 2D-echo in 94% of patients who subsequently developed MI; 84% of patients without acute MI had normal wall motion on the initial 2D-echo[2]. Such segmental wall motion abnormalities are observed in both transmural and nontransmural MI; the incidence in patients with subendocardial wall MI ranges from 83 to 100%.[2-4] Regional akinesis or dyskinesis usually signifies transmural infarction while normal segmental wall motion excludes transmural infarction. Subendocardial wall injury usually produces less profound wall motion abnormalities (hypokinesis) and may occasionally be associated with normal segmental wall motion.[5]

Asynergy outside the electrocardiographic infarct zone is frequently observed during acute MI and is most commonly seen in patients with significant multivessel coronary obstruction[4,6]. Increased oxygen demand on this noninfarcted but hypoperfused myocardium may result in "ischemia at a distance" and consequently abnormal regional wall motion.[4] In contrast, a compensatory hyperkinesis of the noninfarcted wall is usually seen in patients with only one vessel coronary disease.[6]

Expansion of infarction defined as regional dilation, recognized pathologically as stretching and thinning of the infarct zone, can occur within days of acute transmural MI and be identified by 2D-echocardiography.[7] Expansion should be distinguished from infarction extension which implies new myocardial necrosis and can occur in approximately 25 to 50% of patients 4-5 days after hospital admission.[8]

Apart from regional wall motion abnormalities, echocardiography may frequently demonstrate abnormal systolic thickening or even thinning of the involved wall in acute MI.[9] Although quantification of the infarcted myocardium appears promising in experimental animals utilizing various techniques (contrast-enhanced echocardiography, digitized calculation of wall thickening and/or wall motion) only semi-quantitative methods have been utilized to estimate the extent of myocardial involvement in patients with acute MI. According to these methods a wall motion index or score is obtained by dividing the left ventricular wall in several segments. (See Figure 1) These echocardiographic estimates of infarct size correlated well with the extent of infarction assessed by creatine-kinase isoenzyme (CK-MB) measurements[10] and thallium-201 perfusion scan or technetium-99m pyrophosphate scintigraphy.[11] Correlation of

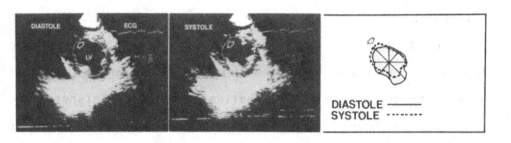

FIGURE 1. Two-dimensional echocardiographic short axis view of the left ventricle (LV) during DIASTOLE, and SYSTOLE and schematic diagram (right panel) showing septal dyskinesis (arrowheads) and hypokinesis of the anterolateral wall in a patient with acute anterior wall myocardial infarction. The left ventricle is divided in 8 segments (right panel) for the semi-quantitative estimation of extent of infarction.
ECG = electrocardiogram

extent of myocardial injury assessed by 2D-echo with pathologic estimations showed a close correlation of the circumferential extent of akinesis/dyskinesis and circumferential extent of scar.[5] Echocardiography somewhat overestimated the actual amount of infarcted myocardium. Regional wall motion abnormalities adjacent to scar or reversibly ischemic areas in the distribution of a significantly obstructed coronary artery may explain this difference.[5]

Thus 2D-echo is a useful noninvasive technique for the immediate diagnosis or exclusion of acute MI and can be performed serially to assess segmental function of both the infarcted and uninvolved regions. More precise means of quantification of infarct size by 2D-echo are under investigation.

COMPLICATIONS OF ACUTE MI:

Papillary muscle dysfunction or rupture

Ischemia or infarction of the papillary muscles, especially of the postero-medial papillary muscle is not uncommon in patients with coronary artery disease and may be associated with variable degrees of mitral regurgitation.[12] Papillary muscle dysfunction is usually seen in patients with inferior wall MI and/or significant right coronary artery obstruction and in patients with left ventricular dilatation or aneurysm. The involved papillary muscle may apear on 2D-echo more dense due to fibrosis and the attached mitral valve leaflet may be displaced apically and held in a rigid position.[13]

Papillary muscle rupture is uncommon, occurring in about 1% of patients 1 to 30 days after an acute MI (inferior wall MI in the majority of cases).[14] Rupture of an entire papillary muscle is usually fatal. Most patients who survive the acute event have rupture of only one or two heads of one of the papillary muscles, most commonly the posteromedial, and present with acute severe mitral regurgitation and intractable pulmonary edema.[12,13] A flail mitral valve is usually detected by 2D-echo in these patients associated with left ventricular enlargement and exaggerated septal motion but decreased motion of the posterior wall. The actual ruptured site and part of the papillary muscle may occasionally be identified. Immediate diagnosis and surgical intervention can be life-saving when this complication occurs.[14]

Ventricular Septal Rupture

Rupture of ventricular septum occurs in 1% of patients with acute MI of either inferior or anterior wall.[13,15] Two dimensional echocardiography may permit direct visualization of the septal defect, which tends to occur at the center of a septal aneurysm and is commonly associated with akinesis or dyskinesis of the interventricular septum.[12,16] Multiple and off-axis views are required to maximize detection of the septal defect. Contrast echocardiography with a negative contrast effect in the right ventricle or a positive contrast effect in the left ventricle may confirm the presence or detect an unsuspected septal defect.[16] Since ventricular septal rupture after acute MI is clinically indistinguishable from papillary muscle rupture, 2D-echo can be useful in recognizing the cause of acute hemodynamic deterioration and allowing early surgery.

Left ventricular aneurysm and thrombus

The incidence of true left ventricular aneurysm after MI ranges from 4-20% in autopsy studies and usually involves the apical left ventricular wall.[12] Patients with ventricular aneurysm often develop thrombi. In one study[17] thrombi were detected by 2D-echo an average of 5 days after the infarction (range 1-11 days) in 46% of patients with apical akinesis or dyskinesis. Patients with inferior MI or anterior infarction without a severe apical wall motion abnormality appear to be at low risk for the development of thrombus.

Myocardial wall rupture

Small amounts of pericardial effusion may be present in patients with post-infarction pericarditis. Large effusions and pericardial tamponade, however, are usually the results of complete left ventricular wall rupture which may occur within the first 10 days after transmural infarction and is associated with poor outcome.[12] Incomplete rupture of the myocardial wall occurring in less than 1% of patients with acute MI may result in pseudoaneurysm. False left ventricular aneurysm or pseudoaneurysm forms at the site of ventricular rupture as a distented, thin-walled sac which frequently contains organized thrombus.[18] Two dimensional echocardiography can differentiate pseudoaneurysm from true left ventricular aneurysm; in pseudoaneurysm the neck or orifice connecting it with the left ventricle is narrow and usually less than the total diameter of the aneurysmal sac.[18] In contrast to true aneurysm, pseudoaneurysms are prone to fatal complete rupture and usually require surgical correction.

Right ventricular infarction

Regional wall motion abnormalities of the free or diaphragmatic wall of the right ventricle can be detected by 2D-echo in patients with right ventricular infarction, which is invariably associated with inferior MI.[19] It is clinically important to recognize right ventricular infarction since fluid administration and avoidance of diuretics are essential to management. Furthermore, 2D-echo can be helpful in excluding the presence of pericardial tamponade, constrictive pericarditis and restrictive cardiomyopathy, conditions with similar clinical and hemodynamic features with right ventricular infarction.[20]

DETERMINTION OF PROGNOSIS IN ACUTE MYOCARDIAL INFARCTION:

Pathologic and clinical evidence suggests that the quantity and location of infarcted or ischemic myocardium are directly related to the morbidity and mortality associated with acute MI. Semi-quantitative 2D-echo methods for the estimation of extent of MI utilized a wall motion index for the overall assessment of left ventricular asynergy.[21,22] (Figure 1)

Patients with uncomplicated infarction usually have a lower wall motion index or score compared to patients with post-infarction in-hospital complications (pulmonary congestion, peripheral hypoperfusion or death).[21,22] In addition severe wall motion abnormalities outside the infarct zone correlated with a greater prevalence of death, cardiogenic shock and reinfarction after the acute infarction.[4] Whether 2D-echo performed during the acute phase of MI can also predict the long-term prognosis is not yet known. In one study[23] patients with infarct expansion detected by 2D-echo within 3 weeks of transmural infarction had more impaired functional status during long-term follow-up (over 3 to 30 month period).

CONCLUSION:

Two dimensional echocardiography is a noninvasive, relative inexpensive technique which can easily be performed at the bedside even in critically ill patients with acute MI. Technically optimal studies in this setting can be obtained in 70-90% of patients.[1,2] Compared to other imaging techniques, 2D-echo offers distinct advantages for evaluating myocardial structure and function in acute MI as well as examine the pericardium and the function of cardiac valves. Thus, it can be used for the immediate diagnosis of acute MI in patients with non-diagnostic electrocardiographic changes and possibly in screening patients admitted with the chest pain syndrome. A clinically or electrocardiographically silent previous MI is a limitation in diagnosing a new infarction by 2D-echo. Serial echocardiographic studies can be performed to assess the functional status of the noninfarcted myocardium and detect the development of expansion or extension of myocardial infarction. In patients with a new systolic murmur or unexplained congestive failure and hypotension after acute MI, 2D-echo can identify the cause and detect possible mechanical complications thus guiding the appropriate medical or surgical intervention. Finally, semi-quantitative wall motion indices of left ventricular asynergy after acute MI can be used to predict the short-term and possibly the long-term prognosis of these patients.

TABLE I

ECHOCARDIOGRAPHY IN ACUTE MYOCARDIAL INFARCTION (MI)

1. Immediate diagnosis:

   a) Regional wall motion abnormalities

      - transmural MI
      - Subendocardial MI

   b) Detection of infarction expansion, extension and distant ischemia

   c) Screening patients with chest pain syndrome

   d) Semi-quantitative estimation of infarct size

2. Detection of Complications:

   a) Dysfunction or rupture of papillary muscles

   b) Ventricular septal rupture

   c) Myocardial wall rupture

      - incomplete (pseudoaneurysm)
      - complete (pericardial effusion and tamponade)

   d) True ventricular aneurysm

   e) Left ventricular thrombus

   f) Right ventricular infarction

3. Determination of Prognosis:

   a) Short term (in-hospital congestive heart failure, cardiogenic shock, death)

   b) ? Long term

BIBLIOGRAPHY

1. Heger JJ, Weyman AE, Wann LS, Dillon JC, Feigenbaum H: Cross-sectional Echocardiography in Acute Myocardial Infarction: Detection and Localization of Regional Left Ventricular Asynergy, Circulation 60:531-538, 1979.

2. Horowitz RS, Morganroth J, Parrotto C, Chen CC, Soffer J, and Pauletto FJ. Immediate Diagnosis of Acute Myocardial Infarction by Two-dimensional Echocardiography, Circulation 65:323-329, 1982.

3. Loh, IK, Charuzi Y, Beeder C, Marshall LA, Ginsburg JH, Early Diagnosis of Nontransmural Myocardial Infarctin by Two-dimensional Echocardiography, Am Heart J 104: 963-968, 1982.

4. Gibson RS, Bishop HL, Stamm RB, Crampton RS, Beller GA, Martin RP. Value of Early Two Dimensional Echocardiography in Patients With Acute Myocardial Infarction, Am J Cardiol 49:1110-1119, 1982.

5. Weiss JL, Bulkley BH, Hutchins GM, Mason SJ. Two-dimensional Echocardiographic Recognition of Myocardial Injury in Man: Comparison with Postmortem Studies, Circulation 63:401-408, 1981.

6. Stamm RB, Gibson RS, Bishop HL, Carabello BA, Beller GA, Martin RP, Echocardiographic detection of infarct-localized asynergy and remote asynergy during acute myocardial infarction: Correlation with the extent of angiographic coronary disease, Circulation 67:233-244, 1983.

7. Eaton LW, Weiss JL, Bulkley BH, Garrison JB, Weisfeldt ML, Regional Cardiac Dilatation After Acute Myocardial Infarction: Recognition by Two-dimensional Echocardiography, N Engl J Med 300:57-62, 1979.

8. Willerson JT: Echocardiography After Acute Myocardial Infarction, N Engl J Med 300:87-89. (Editorial)

9. Corya BC, Rasmussen S, Feigenbaum H, Knoebel SB, Black MJ, Systolic Thickening and Thinning of the Septum and Posterior Wall in Patients with Coronary Artery Disease, Congestive Cardiomyopathy, and Atrial Septal Defect, Circulation 55:109-14, 1977.

10. Visser CA, Lie KI, Kan G, Meltzer R, Durrer D, Detection and Quantification of Acute Isolated Myocardial Infarction by Two-dimensional Echocardiography, Am J Cardiol 47:1020-5, 1981.

11. Nixon JV, Narahara KA, Smitherman TC, Estimation of Myocardial involvement in patients with acute myocardial Infarction by Two-dimensional Echocardiography. Circulation 62:1248-55, 1980.

12. Kotler MN, Mintz GS, Segal BL, Operable Complications of MI: Noninvasive Diagnosis, J of Cardiovas Med, 7:1070-1077, 1982.

13. Mintz GS, Victor MF, Kotler MN, Parry WR, Segal BL, Two-dimensional Echocardiographic Identification of Surgically Correctable Complications of Acute Myocardial Infarction. Circulation 64:91-96, 1981.

14. Nishimura RA, Schaff HV, Shub C, Gersh BJ, Edwards WB, Tajik AJ, Papillary Muscle Rupture Complicating Acute Myocardial Infarction: Analysis of 17 patients, Am J Cardiol 51:373-7, 1983.

15. Bishop HL, Gibson RS, Stamm RB, Beller GA, Martin RP, Role of Two-dimensional echocardiography in the Evaluation of Patients with Ventricular Septal Rupture Postmyocardial Infarction, Am Heart J, 102:965-71, 1981.

16. Drobac M, Gilbert B, Howard R, Baigrie R, Rakowski H, Ventricular Septal Defect After Myocardial Infarction: Diagnosis by Two-dimensional Contrast Echocardiography, Circulation 67:335-341, 1983.

17. Asinger RW, Mikell FL, Elsperger J, Hodges M, Incidence of Left-Ventricular Thrombosis After Acute Transmural Myocardial Infaraction. Serial Evaluation by Two-dimensional Echocardiography, N Engl J Med, 305:297-302, 1981.

18. Catherwood E, Mintz GS, Kotler MN, Parry WR, Segal BL, Two-dimensional Echocardiographic Recognition of Left Ventricular Pseudoaneurysm, Circulation 62:294-303, 1980.

19. D'Arcy B, Nanda NC, Two-dimensional Echocardiograhic Features of Right Ventricular Infarction, Circulation 65:167-73, 1982.

20. Lorell B, Leinbach RC, Pohost GM, Gold HK, Dinsmore RE, Hutter AM Jr, Pastore JO, Desanctis RW, Right Ventricular Infarction. Clinical Diagnosis and Differentiation from Cardiac Tamponade and Pericardial Constriction, Am J Cardiol 43:465-71, 1979.

21. Heger JJ, Weyman AE, Wann LS, Rogers EW, Dillion JC, Feigenbaum H, Cross-sectional Echocardiographic Analysis of the Extent of Left Ventricular Asynergy in Acute Myocardial Infarction, Circulation 61:1113-1118, 1980.

22. Horowitz RS, Morganroth J: Immediate Detection of Early High-Risk Patients with Acute Myocardial Infarction Using Two-Dimensional Echocardiographic Evaluation of Left Ventricular Regional Wall Motion Abnormalities, Am Heart J 103:814-822, 1982.

23. Erlebacher JA, Weiss JL, Eaton LW, Kallman C, Weisfeldt ML, Bulkley BH, Late Effects of Acute Infarct Dilation on Heart Size: A Two Dimensional Echocardiographic Study, Am J Cardiol, 49:1120-1126, 1982.

9

PANEL ON INDICES TO DEFINE INFARCT SIZE

Moderator: Dr. Joel Morganroth

Dr. Morganroth: If one had to offer advice on the preferred method of studying an intervention in patients with acute myocardial infarction to determine whether that intervention was affecting the extent of the damage from myocardial infarction and if this intervention was used in a large, multicenter clinical trial, rather than a single institution, what would be your thoughts as to the best end points to study?

Dr. Sobel: To answer this question one would have to know what the intervention was to be looked at. For instance, let's say that we had an intervention that among other things chewed up enzymes and if you wanted to study that intervention and you used enzymes as your end point, they would be meaningless. If you had another intervention, that didn't happen to do that, you might get a good answer. If one wanted to study the effect of something on the anatomy of the heart, let's say expansion, I might want to use nuclear magnetic resonance for that because the anatomical imaging is so powerful or I might want to use gated CT scanning because the resolution is so good. But if I were interested in a different question, that wasn't quite so highly focused and so very specific, I might want to use something that had much more universal applicability, and the enzyme curves as I tried to point out are very useful in that sense, if the intervention that is being studied has been shown conclusively, not to distort the curves in an unpredictable way. So in the case of thrombolysis if you took the curves and interpreted them the way we did for other types of studies, you would be mislead, but it may well be that with experimental laboratory information that is coming from many centers now, we will be able to interpret those curves unambiguously and they would be very useful in large trials as they have been in the European cooperative trial where they have been useful for dating the onset of reperfusion, the frequency of reperfusion in the patients studied, and in fact the apparent effect on infarct size. It has been shown that with thrombolytic therapy in patients

when reperfusion was successful, even though the peak CK values were higher
and the rate of upstroke of the curve was more rapid than in the
non-reperfused people, the areas under the curves were smaller so they could
see the apparent benefit of salvage induced that way using the enzymes. I
think what the question points to is that the end point has to be very closely
married to the question being posed in a clinical trial and that undoubtedly,
most trials will require more than one end point because more than one question is really being asked.

Dr. Morganroth: While I agree that there are some interventions that might
eliminate a particular end point measurement, I think your answer to my
question was that the enzymatic approach would be a reasonable generally
applicable technique as a particular end point in an intervention trial. Dr.
Willerson, is that the only technique that you would use for advice in terms
of multi-center national cooperative trials? Would you use just enzymatic or
would you add some other measure, such as a noninvasive technique?

Dr. Willerson: I agree with Dr. Sobel's thoughtful answer to the question. However, I would want to make some measurement of global and segmental
function. I might pick a different measure of infarct size, but it would
depend on the question asked and problem studied. I think that ultimately one
has to know about the preservation of at least segmental function and its
contribution to global ventricular function with any index of infarct size.
The whole rationale that we use is that one of these measurements which
identifies the smaller infarct size would be associated with better preserved
ventricular function and a longer life, a better quality life; a life without
so many symptoms related to a large infarct.

Dr. Morganroth: Would radionuclide left ventricular ejection fraction be a
useful measure in that regard, or is there a better index?

Dr. Willerson: I think there probably is a better index of global
function. I think that the smallest volume that the heart can contract down
to the end systolic volume, is less influenced by preload and heart rate
and if measured at the right time probably several weeks after a hopefully
favorable intervention. If you think about thrombolytic therapy and measure

the impact of that on ventricular segmental or global function, within the first few hours, days or probably the first week after the event, you really don't provide the opportunity to look at the full restoration of function. In the animal model that requires somewhere between two weeks and a month. At rest, I don't know why 2-D echocardiography or ultimately NMR imaging should also be excellent means to look at the same problem.

Dr. Moore: One concern that I have and that I am sure that many others have is that the Federal Government is going to have Medicare and Medicaid pay only a certain number of dollars for a given procedure. That is, if a person has an infarct, there is going to be only a certain number of dollars paid to take care of that person. I think this is going to slow some of these very expensive techniques. It emphasizes that private industry is going to have to pick up a number of these innovative ways to actually predict further damage and to predict the size of the damage during clinical studies. Do any of the clinicians have any comments on what the effect of this is going to be made on the advances that are made in these very sophisticated techniques?

Dr. Reimer: I have a comment on another aspect.' I would like to stress the importance of post mortem anatomic studies in clinical trials on interventions on infarct size and quite clearly, most post-mortem studies are not going to be a primary end point, because most of the patients are going to hopefully survive and and the information will not be available. I think from the point of view of continuing ongoing quality control, we need to look at a select number of patients, those that are dying in order to evaluate how good the various clinical indices are in the particular study and this is particularly important along the lines of what Dr. Sobel brought up, that the intervention itself may influence the clinical index used to estimate infarct size. I think anatomic studies are often unfortunately left out of planning of clinical trials.

Dr. Sobel: I would like to come back to Dr. Moore's question, because I think it is a very critical question and I think the real answer to it, is that the clinicians functioning in their patient care capacities are going to stop doing a lot of things of equivocal value in patient care but which may be very valuable in clinical research. I think that is appropriate. I think there has been in cardiology, a natural inclination to fall in love with technology because it is so terribly exciting and for things that could be

justified well as research enterprises to spill into clinical practice with
some lack of discrimination. I think the net effect on patient care initially
will not be bad because the physician is very able to discriminate about which
test he needs to make, which management decision. The net effect on research
which you allude to should be zero, but unfortunately won't be zero. It
should be zero because we should not be using clinical practice environments
to support research. We should be supporting researchers' research. In fact,
in most prestigious institutions, that is the case, but in many institutions
in which research capability is not as easily acquired from the NIH or
industry, unfortunately, if the truth be known, there are things billed to
patients occasionally that are not simply dictated by practice and I think
that that will have to stop because the government and third party carriers
aren't going to reimburse and the patients will probably rebel. If the
research establishment supports the development of the technologies in which
we are interested for research reasons, then the impact will not be negative
on investigation, but the impact will be perhaps positive on reducing practice
costs and making the physician much more discriminating about what he wants to
take into the practice armamentarium in any given point in time. Related to
that, I really want to underscore, that my feelings about using enzymes in
large scale clinical trials are not in any sense exclusive. I certainly don't
believe that one cannot look at the function of the ventricle, or the health
of the patient, or the survival of the patient, or the morphology of the heart
in those who die, but I was in trying to answer that question in part in terms
of economics of large scale clinical trials. There are some trials in which
very expensive end points have been used in which we learn during the course
of the trial that the end point was ambiguous. A good example would be global
ejection fraction with thrombolysis in which the compensatory segment behaved
in the opposite way and as a result, you saw the wrong directional change in
ejectional fraction even though segmental wall motion was improved by
reperfusion in a consistent fashion. That was a critical investigation of far
reaching implications for all of us that want to use nuclear medicine
techniques or ventricular graphic techniques to assess what is happening. We
have to look at the segment involved. We can't simply look at a global
measure. Now the global measure is important because if the patient has
really benefitted and his ejection fraction is low, he would be better off.
But none of these things should be viewed as exclusive and in the case of the
question that Dr. Moore raised, I think we have to make a clear distinction

between clinical practice and what these new regulations are going to do to that and clinical research.

Dr. Ruberio: Dr. Reimer, you showed a nice correlation between measuring the collateral flow and infarct size. In your slide you showed that you are measuring the flow post therapy. I was wondering that if you give a beneficial intervention that alters the coronary collateral circulation which alters your evaluation technique can you show any pharmacological beneficial intervention reduce infarct size.

Dr. Reimer: The one way that you can measure of collateral blood flow with an intervention, is to measure collateral blood flow immediately after occlusion and then begin your intervention and then measure collateral blood flow at a later point after the intervention has occurred. Then you can observe the effect of the intervention per se on collateral blood flow and you can also observe the relationship between the collateral blood and infarct size using both the collateral blood flow measured before the intervention and that measured after the intervention.

Dr. Ruberio: In using this technique were you able to demonstrate any beneficial pharmacological intervention reducing infarct size?

Dr. Reimer: We have not studied that many different interventions, but the answer is that we have not shown a beneficial effect with verapamil, propranolol or with hyaluronidase.

Dr. Ruberio: Dr. Sobel, I would like to ask you about what you think about the mitochondrial creatinokinase that you started developing some time ago and claim that it would detect irreversible necrosis. Where does it stand at the moment?

Dr. Sobel: That work is Dr. Bob Roberts' work. We developed jointly a radioaminoassay for mitochondrial CK. He then went on to show that in experimental animals, the mitochondrial enzyme appeared in the plasma at about the same time as the conventional cytoplasmic isozyme forms, but that it had a very short half life and his hope was that this would permit a kind of staccato dating of repetitive injury. When he wrote the paper in which he said that it might have some value in distinguishing irreversible from reversible injury, I protested since Carmen showed in the 50's and others that cells subjected to ischemia don't release macromolecules unless they are dead. You can get a cell to do that under other circumstances, but not under circumstances of ischemia. So as far as I am concerned personally, there is no difference in the implication of release of mitochondrial enzyme as opposed to cycto enzyme. I can't imagine an insult due to ischemia that will hurt the cell sufficiently that it will break its membrane and the mitochondria stay happy and it rejuventates. I think you could make that happen in an artificial setting with calcium deprivation or various other things. But in man, when we have coronary blood flow interruptions if it is bad enough to rupture the sarcolema, that is enough and the cell is going to die. The value clinically of mitochondrial CK determinations may include more precise dating of the episodic onset of injury cause of half times, it may include some sensitivity issues that conceivably could be addressed. I don't think it will be very useful in differentiating reversible from irreversible injury.

Dr.Sleight: I would like to ask the panel about the question of when you can intervene in acute infarction. Dr. Sobel showed very persuasively with the animal models that he was looking at 2 hours and that was about it. It would seem logical that if you used for instance streptokinase that you have got to get in in that time. But on the other hand, when you analyze the publications in man as to the benefit from streptokinase then it seems that it is not absolutely as clear cut as that and particularly as you know there is some evidence that you can get benefit later, perhaps when in people with better collaterals. I would like some views on that and the last point I would like to make is about fibrinogen which has just been mentioned. It might seem bad to reduce your fibrinogen and you bleed, but on the other hand it might have some beneficial effects on viscosity. It is a sort of multi-barreled question, but it is to do with the timing of intervention.

Dr. Willerson: In animal models it does seem clear that one cannot wait longer than about 4 hours after coronary occlusion (and probably better two or three hours) to obtain reflow and get some protection of segmental function. There is rather uniform agreement about that when sensitive methods have been used. That is reperfusion by itself. It really does not address the question as to whether reperfusion plus some effective pharmacologic intervention might

expand this window. It might allow a longer time period of salvage of
jeopardized myocardium and allow one to intervene later with reperfusion.
Really, I think that was the rationale on which Maroko and Braunwald developed
the idea that pharmacologic intervention might protect ischemic myocardium,
understanding that somehow new blood flow would have to be brought to the
ischemic area and that one might be able to temporize with some intervention
or set of interventions. Unfortunately, efforts immediately became focused on
permanent coronary artery occlusion and in that setting, one can't do very
much for a very long period of time. I think we should look forward to
studies that couple reperfusion with effective pharmacologic intervention,
intervention that might decrease metabolic requirements, might decrease oxygen
demand, might reduce calcium uptake in injured myocardium, might protect cells
directly and their membranes, might delay the activation of certain enzymes,
lysosomal and other enzyme systems, and the damaged membranes and cells
directly and really asks the question in the forseeable future, would some
combination of interventions with reperfusion, at the outset be protective. I
think we will just have to wait to see about that. I wouldn't be terribly
pessimistic about it. I think some extension of this window with appropriate
pharmacologic intervention may be possible. In man it is hard to date the
time of infarction. I think that is one problem that might explain some of
the discrepant results. Certainly there are patients who have collateral
perfusion, smaller or larger infarcts, hypertrophy or not, have been on
certain protective interventions chronically and they are continued and even
in some of the clinical studies have waited up to 18 hours after infarction
and get some recovery. But a number of different pharmacologic interventions
have been used in those studies. Some of those patients have stuttering and
continuing chest pain, not one episode of pain, but rather ongoing infarction
or very delayed infarction even though it seems to be relatively old. I think
all of those are formidable problems for interpreting what one does in man in
terms of the time of reperfusion it might be protective. It is easier to study
in animal models.

Dr. Moore: I wanted to make a comment regarding the electrical stability of
the heart following maintained total occlusion versus reperfusion after total
occlusion of two hours. It has been well known for many years that if one
totally occludes the left anterior descending coronary artery and leaves that
total occlusion on, then the spontaneous arrhythmias are over in about 72

hours. Also with total occlusion models, one cannot induce arrhythmias with programmed electrical stimulation beyond about 7 days. However, if you occlude permanently for two hours and then you allow total reperfusion to continue, one gets a very different type of infarct than with total continuous occlusion. In the two hour occlusion with reperfusion infarct model, you get a heterogeneous "swiss cheese" type infarct and those hearts are very electrically unstable. Programmed electrical stimulation can reproducibly start tachyarrhythmias in that model. Our group has studied dogs who have undergone two hours of occlusion followed by reperfusion and even at 2 years, these dogs can with programmed electrical stimulation be put into tachyarrhthmias. So if you reperfuse after two hours, you may be causing a heart to become more electrically unstable than if you allow that total occlusion to be maintained.

Dr.Goldstein: There seems to be a contradiction, in terms of Dr. Reimer's position and Dr. Sobel's position on enzyme release, which is perplexing to me. One is that enzymes are only released in dead cells, yet Dr. Reimer shows very elegantly that if one does establish reflow within 3 hours one can or at least certainly with a few hours, one can return the cell to at least anatomic normality. Is it possible that one could release enzymes and still have a normal cell that could be revived.

Dr. Sobel: Dr. Goldstein, I don't think there is any disagreement at all particularly since Dr. Reimer is the only morphologist to ever prove unequivocally that CK enzyme curves worked. I am very grateful to him. I think what we are both saying is that in any model, there is a time when some of the cells in the jeopardized region are not yet dead. Those particular cells would not have released their enzyme constituents into the blood, but the cell next door may well be dead and it would have. Now if you reperfuse, that cell that wasn't quite dead and didn't contribute to the enzyme release will potentially be salvageable. I don't think we disagree at all on that point unless I am mistaken.

I also wanted to answer the rest of Dr. Sleight's question about fibrinogen. I think the real answer is that it is a matter of how much. It is like being a little pregnant. If the fibrinogen is modestly diminished and FDP's accumulated don't cause massive bleeding don't cause a DIC syndrome, the viscosity is indeed lowered as you rightly pointed out and that will facilitate an improvement in ejection fraction which incidently may account for some of these marvelous late effects that we have been snookered into getting excited about, perhaps inappropriately, but no one will argue that if you take all the fibrinogen away that the patient is a set-up for a disaster. It undoubtedly is a matter of degree and duration of impairment with the coagulation system and all of its ramifications. Fibrinogen is only one of the elements that I happened to focus on but one could take this to a lot of other aspects of the system. Just to complete the loop, I agree very completely with what Jim said. The reason for my emphasizing the time in animals was to sort of define some limits. In human beings I happen to believe that the stuttering infarct is probably routine and once a patient is transiently impaired, functionally he is likely to have limited perfusion into some other areas near fixed obstructions or perhaps even alterations in tone and that over a period of many hours, he sustains a whole host of little infarcts. The reason that you got such very nice results in your own clinical studies with beta blockers, is that I think you prevented part of the stuttering infarct, and that we have a larger window to work with in man for many reasons than we are likely to have in animals where we ligate something or put a catheter or make a massive clot.

Dr. Willerson: We have a larger window in some patients and not in others and it is extremely variable.

Dr. Morganroth: I think this panel discussion has pointed out that there is a wide variety of facts yet to be determined that are quite critical in even planning the simplest clinical trial. The end points to use will not only depend on the intervention, but will depend on the availability of the variety of methods available to measure what is happening to the heart, either enzymatically, electrophysiologically, or to segmental wall motion by nuclear or echocardiographic techniques.

10

THE CASE FOR PROPHYLACTIC LIDOCAINE IN ACUTE MYOCARDIAL INFARCTION

DONALD C. HARRISON, M.D.

INTRODUCTION

Although lidocaine has been widely used for the treatment of ventricular arrhythmias for more than two decades, its routine prophylactic administration after acute myocardial infarction remains controversial (1,2). Numerous animal studies and studies in man have demonstrated that lidocaine elevates the threshold for ventricular fibrillation and is highly effective in abolishing ventricular arrhythmias after acute myocardial infarction (1,3-8). Since other less serious ventricular arrhythmias were noted before ventricular fibrillation in many instances, a seemingly rational program for the administration of lidocaine to suppress these so-called warning arrhythmias which hearlded ventricular fibrillation in acute myocardial infarction was developed (9-11). In addition, lidocaine had been proposed for pre-hospital administration to prevent sudden death in patients experiencing myocardial infarction during transport to the hospital (12,13).

Because of the frequent use of lidocaine in patients with acute myocardial infarction and the possible application of the drug to reduce the incidence of sudden death in the early period after acute myocardial infarction, the concept of its routine prophylactic administration has been developed (1,2,14,9). The purpose of this review is to outline the basis for proposing the administration of lidocaine prophylactically in patients with acute myocardial infarction.

EFFECTIVENESS OF LIDOCAINE IN VENTRICULAR ARRHYTHMIAS

Many studies have demonstrated the effectiveness of lidocaine in reducing ventricular ectopic beats and more complex forms of ventricular rhythms in patients experiencing acute myocardial infarction (15-17). In the 1960's, this information led to recommending lidocaine for treating rhythm disturbances which were considered premonitory to sustained ventricular tachycardia (so called "warning arrhythmias") and ventricular fibrillation (9). Thus lidocaine was recommended for premonitory arrhythmias consisting of greater than five premature ventricular contractions per minute or coupled premature ventricular contractions, multiformed premature ventricular contractions, runs of greater than 3 premature ventricular contractions and in any patient who was resuscitated from ventricular tachycardia or ventricular fibrillation (9). These rhythms were considered premonitory to catastrophic rhythm disturbances in patients seen within 24 hours of acute infarction. Subsequently, numerous studies demonstrated that from 25-50% of patients developing ventricular tachycardia or ventricular fibrillation did not experience these premonitory arrhythmias (18,19). While several studies have confirmed these observations, other investigators continue to propose this as a rational basis for lidocaine administration (21).

The available data suggest that lidocaine is highly effective in treating and preventing ventricular ectopic beats in patients with acute myocardial infarction. Recently, the relationship of lidocaine treatment producing a reduction in ectopic beats to the occurrence of ventricular fibrillation was reviewed extensively (21). Considerable heterogenity of patient selection occurred in the sixteen reported studies (21). When the best studies with the largest groups and the greatest patient homogenity were pooled, the effect of lidocaine in preventing ventricular fibrillation was confirmed. In one study by Lie et al (22), a highly statistically significant effect of lidocaine for preventing ventricular fibrillation in a blinded randomized control study was documented. This study (22) has been subjected to many criticisms and the frequent incidence of side effects with high levels of lidocaine being administered has been used to negate the observations of the study. Although there is still reason for controversy, in my opinion, the best evidence suggests that lidocaine is highly effective in reducing ventricular arrhythmias in patients with acute myocardial infarction and in preventing ventricular fibrillation when administered within the first twenty-four hours after infarction.

DETECTION OF PREMONITORY ARRHYTHMIAS

For those investigators who still believe that premonitory arrhythmias hearld the occurrence of sustained ventricular tachycardia or ventricular fibrillation, the question of how frequently these arrhythmias are detected in the average coronary care unit is of interest. Several studies have demonstrated that significant events, that is the occurrence of premonitory arrhythmias, are frequently not detected in the best of coronary care units (23-25). Even with the use of computer-assisted monitoring, a significant number of events are not detected and the delay in administering treatment is highly variable (23). Thus, even if premonitory arrhythmias occur, in the average coronary care unit they are frequently not detected and the administration of lidocaine only to treat such premonitory arrhythmias and thereby preventing ventricular fibrillation, is not a rational approach.

PROGNOSIS AFTER VENTRICULAR FIBRILLATION

Some investigators accept the hypothesis that lidocaine prevents significant episodes of ventricular fibrillation, but do not believe that the occurrence of primary ventricular fibrillation (ventricular fibrillation in the absence of heart failure or cardio-genic shock) alters the prognosis from acute myocardial infarction when it occurs in a well-staffed coronary care unit (26,27). Thus, these investigators suggest careful monitoring of patients and quick and early resuscitation of those experiencing ventricular fibrillation.

On the other hand, Conley and associates (28) followed a group of patients from the coronary care unit for five years and demonstrated a reduced life survival for those having ventricular fibrillation as compared with those who did not. In addition, numbers of patients who experienced primary ventricular fibrillation will not be resuscitated even in the best of coronary care units. Available evidence to date suggests that the prognosis for patients experiencing primary ventricular fibrillation is poorer than those who do not experience ventricular fibrillation. We postulate that in resuscitation potentially viable marginally profused myocardium is lost resulting in a larger infarct size in those patients having ventricular fibrillation. Thus, ventricular fibrillation should not be allowed to occur if the long-term prognosis is to be optimal.

SAFETY FOR LIDOCAINE ADMINISTRATION

In recent years the pharmacokinetics and pharmacodynamics of lidocaine administration has been studied extensively (16, 29, 30). Its use in patients with disease-altered disposition patterns is well understood and a rational program for its administration has been established. In our own coronary care unit, there have been no episodes in the past two years of convulsions due to high levels of lidocaine. Techniques for monitoring blood levels of lidocaine and Bayssian techniques for predicting what levels will be established with an infusion program of administration are available and can be used. The effects of reductions in hepatic blood flow due to lowered cardiac output in patients with heart failure and shock are well understood (31). In these instances, the measurement of plasma levels is helpful in determining steady-state lidocaine levels necessary to maintain antiarrhythmic effects while preventing the occurrence of toxicity. Other side effects such as nausea and vomiting, CNS depression, numbness and tingling of extremities occur frequently with lidocaine but are seldom serious enough to require its discontinuation. Thus, the pharmacokinetics of lidocaine are well enough known to recommend rational prophylactic administration in all patients suffering from acute myocardial infarction.

RECOMMENDATIONS FOR LIDOCAINE ADMINISTRATION

Based upon the arguments above, it is our recommendation that lidocaine be administered prophylactically once the physician has a full understanding of the pharmacology of the drug. We recommend the following program:

1. For all patients admitted to the coronary care unit with a myocardial infarction or a high likelihood of myocardial infarction, prophylactic lidocaine be adminis-

tered for 36-48 hours.

2. In order to achieve an early therapeutic level, a loading dose of 225 mg should be administered over the first thirty minutes together with the simultaneous infusion to 2-3 mg/min by an intravenous route. This loading dose may be given as an initial dose of 100 mg followed by 50 to 75 mg given each 10 minutes during the next thirty minutes. It may also be administered as a 15 mg/min infusion for 15 minutes or as a single loading dose of 225 mg over 30 minutes.

3. Lidocaine should be administered 2-3 mg/min based upon a patient's estimated clearance of the drug. Thus, in patients with low cardiac outputs due to heart failure or cardiogenic shock lower doses might be considered. (We generally recommend 1.0 mg/minute)

4. In patients with altered disposition, lidocaine blood levels should be determined at 4 hours after commencing the drug and at 12 and 24 hours in order to regulate the plasma level to between 1.5 and 5 µg/ml.

5. Lidocaine has been shown to bind to alpha 1 acid glycoproteins (32). These are elevated in patients with acute myocardial infarction after 72 hours, and if the drug is to be administered over a long period of time, free levels of lidocaine should be determined for regulating the dose on a continuing basis.

6. The question of lidocaine's administration in the early period after infarction in regard to its effectiveness has been raised. A number of studies have suggested less effectiveness at the earliest stages after infarction. We believe this to be true since the greatest level of electrical homogeneity occurs during this period of time. However, we believe the drug is generally still effective in most patients. Thus, we believe lidocaine should be administered with a loading dose and continuous intravenous infusion to prevent a therapeutic hiatus occurring at 1-4 hours, and that once steady state conditions are reached, measurement of at least one blood level is important to document that the patient is being maintained in a therapeutic range.

SUMMARY AND CONCLUSION

We recommend the routine prophylactic administration of lidocaine when there is acute myocardial infarction or a high suspicion of acute myocardial infarction. This rationale is based upon our observations and those of others that premonitory arrhythmias do not predict which patients will develop life-threatening catastrophic arrhythmias. Even if such arrhythmias occur and did predict catastrophe, they would frequently be missed by the routine staff of coronary care units. Lidocaine has proven to be effective for the treatment of arrhythmias, and in a number of reasonably well controlled studies shown to reduce the occurrence of ventricular fibrillation. We believe that ventricular fibrillation leads to a poorer prognosis in the five-year follow up after myocardial infarction. Thus every effort should be made to prevent its occurrence.

With new knowledge about pharmacokinetics and pharmacodynamics of lidocaine, a rational program for its administration to all patients can be recommended. Blood level measurements are available in most hospitals and permit monitoring of lidocaine levels to prevent toxicity even in patients with altered dispositions such as those with heart failure, cardiogenic shock, liver disease and renal disease. Thus, our conclusion is that well-trained cardiologists should administer lidocaine prophylactically to patients experiencing acute myocardial infarction.

REFERENCES

1. Berte LE, Harrison DC: Should prophylactic antiarrhythmic drug therapy be employed in acute myocardial infarction? In: SH Rahimtoola (ed) Controversies in coronary artery disease. F.A. Davis Co., Philadelphia, 1982, pp 173-181.
2. Harrison DC: Should lidocaine be administered routinely to all patients after acute myocardial infarction? Circulation (58):581-584, 1978.
3. Harrison DC, Sprouse JH, Morrow AG: Antiarrhythmic properties of lidocaine and procainamide: Clinical and physiologic studies of their cardiovascular effects in man. Circulation (28):486-491, 1963.
4. Singh BN, Vaughn Williams EM: Effects of altering potassium concentration on the actions of lidocaine and diphenylhydration on rabbit atrial and ventricular muscle. Circ Res (29):286-295, 1971.
5. Morgensen L: Ventricular tachyarrhythmias and lignocaine prophylaxis in acute myocardial infarction. A clinical and therapeutic study. Acta Med Scand (513):1-80, 1970.
6. Wyman MG, Hammersmith L: Comprehensive treatment plan for the prevention of primary ventricular fibrillation in acute myocardial infarction. Am J Cardiol (33):661, 1974.
7. Pitt A, Lipp A, Anderston ST: Lignocaine given prophylactically to patients with acute myocardial infarction. Lancet (1):612, 1971.
8. Ribner HS, Isaacs ES, Frishman WH: Lidocaine prophylaxis against ventricular fibrillation in acute myocardial infarction. Prog Cardiovasc Dis (21):287, 1979.
9. Lown B, Fakho AM, Hood WB: The coronary care unit. JAMA (199):188, 1967.
10. Gianelly R, von der Groeben JO, Spivack AP, Harrison DC: Effect of lidocaine on ventricular arrhythmias in patients with coronary artery disease. N Engl J Med (277):1215-1219, 1967.
11. Kostuk WJ, Beanlands DS: The prophylactic use of lidocaine in the prevention of ventricular arrhythmias in acute myocardial infarction. In: Scott DB, Julian DG (ed) Lidocaine in the Treatment of Ventricular Arrhythmias. Livingstone, Edinburgh and London,1971, p 82.
12. Valentine PA, Frew JL, Mashford ML, Sloman GA: Lidocaine in the prevention of sudden death in prehospital phase of acute infarction. N Engl J Med (291):1327, 1974.
13. Pantridge JF: Prehospital coronary care. Br Heart J (26):233, 1974.
14. Harrison DC, Berte LE: Should prophylactic antiarrhythmic drug therapy be used in acute myocardial infarction? JAMA (247):2019-2021, 1982.
15. Alderman EL, Kerber RE, Harrison DC: Evaluation of lidocaine resistance in man using intermittent large-dose infusion techniques. Am J Cardiol (34):342-349, 1974.
16. Harrison DC, Meffin PJ, Winkle RA: Clinical pharmacokinetics of antiarrhythmic drugs. Progr Cardiovasc Dis (20):217-242, 1977.

17. Harrison DC, Alderman EL: The pharmacology and clinical use of lidocaine as an antiarrhythmic drug -- 1972. In: Modern Treatment 9: 1972. Hagerstown, Md, Harper and Row (monograph), pp 139-175.

18. Dhurandhar RW, MacMillan RL, Brown KWG: Primary ventricular fibrillation complicating acute myocardial infarction. Am J Cardiol (27):347, 1971.

19. Lie KI, Wellens HJ, Durrer D: Characteristics and predictability of primary ventricular fibrillation. Eur J Cardiol (1):379, 1974.

20. Lown B: Sudden cardiac death: the major challenge confronting contemporary cardiology. Am J Cardiol (43):313-328, 1979.

21. DeSilva RA, Hennekens CH, Lown B, Casscells W: Lignocaine prophylaxis in acute myocardial infarction: an evaluation of randomised trials. Lancet 855-858, 1981.

22. Lie KI, Wellens JH, van Capelle FJ, Durrer D: Lidocaine in the prevention of primary ventricular fibrillation. A double-blind, randomized study of 212 consecutive patients. N Engl J Med (291):1324, 1974.

23. Romhilt DW, Bloomfield SS, Chou T-C. Fowler NO: Unreliability of conventional electrocardiographic monitoring for arrhythmia detection in coronary care units. Am J Cardiol (31):457, 1973.

24. Holmberg S, Ryden L, Waldenstrom A: Efficiency of arrhythmia detection by nurses in a coronary care unit using a decentralised monitoring system. Br Heart J (39):1019, 1977.

25. Vetter NJ, Julian DG: Comparison of arrhythmia computer and conventional monitoring in coronary-care unit. Lancet (1):1151, 1975.

26. Dupont B, Flensted-Jensen E, Sandoe E: The long-term prognosis for patients resuscitated after cardiac arrest. Am Heart J (78):444, 1969.

27. McNamee B, Robinson T, Adgey A: Long-term prognosis following ventricular fibrillation in acute ischemic heart disease. Br Med J (4):204, 1970.

28. Conley MJ, McNeer JF, Lee KL: Cardiac arrest complicating acute myocardial infarction: Predictibility and prognosis. Am J Cardiol (39):7, 1977.

29. Winkle RA, Glantz SA, Harrison DC: Pharmacologic therapy of ventricular arrhythmias. Am J Cardiol (36):629, 1975.

30. Greenblatt J, Bolognini V, Koch-Weser J: Pharmacokinetic approach to the clinical use of lidocaine intravenously. JAMA (236):273, 1976.

31. Stenson RE, Constantino RT, Harrison DC: Interrelationships of hepatic blood flow, cardiac output, and blood levels of lidocaine in man. Circulation 43:205, 1971.

32. Routledge PA, Stargel WW, Wagner GS, Shand D: Increased alpha-1-acid glyoco-protein and lidocaine disposition in myocardial infarction. Ann Intern Med (93):701, 1980.

11

INFARCT SIZE REDUCTION BY ANTIARRHYTHMIC PROPHYLAXIS - A CONTRARY VIEW.

R.W.F. CAMPBELL, P. KERTES

1.   INTRODUCTION

Acute myocardial infarction is not an instantaneous event and in the first few hours, many important progressive pathophysiologic changes occur. Cell death may take some hours and for a critically short time period from the onset of ischaemia, cellular recovery is possible. Moreover, within the so-called "border zone" of infarction, minor alterations in the relatively precarious balance of oxygen supply and demand may enlarge or restrict the final extent of irreversible damage. Although limitation of infarct size has a reasonable basis in animal experimentation[1] there is a paucity of evidence that meaningful infarct size limitation can be achieved in man.

Whilst studies of beta-adrenoreceptor blocking drugs[2] suggest that they may influence infarct size, there have been few investigations of the effects of non-betablocking antiarrhythmic therapies.

2.   MECHANISMS

There are three mechanisms by which antiarrhythmic therapy might limit infarct size.

2.1   Effect by Antiarrhythmic Action

During the critical time period when myocardial salvage may be possible, clinical acute myocardial infarction frequently is complicated by arrhythmias of which ventricular fibrillation and ventricular tachycardia are the most important[3]. By causing serious haemodynamic upset, both may encourage infarct expansion. Prophylactic antiarrhythmic therapy potentially might have two benefits - prevention of arrhythmias and infarct size limitation although by this mechanism, the latter advantage would acrue only to those patients in whom an arrhythmia was prevented.

2.2   Effects by other than antiarrhythmic action

Antiarrhythmic compounds might limit infarct size by an action unrelated to their antiarrhythmic activity. In non-clinical experiments, a
large range of agents[1] are reported to reduce or limit infarct size
although often the mechanism of action is not fully understood. Animal
studies have revealed that verapamil[4] and lidocaine[5,6,7,8] can reduce
infarct size; the effect being unrelated to a direct antiarrhythmic
action. In man beta-adrenoreceptor blocking drugs[2] appear to reduce
infarct size but there is no evidence that antiarrhythmic drugs of Vaughan
Williams Class I have this effect. The negative inotropic effect of many
membrane-active antiarrhythmic agents might affect infarct size either
beneficially through reduction of myocardial work and improvement of the
oxygen supply-demand ratio, or detrimentally by reducing perfusion of
jeopardised myocardium.

2.3.   Spurious

Antiarrhythmic therapy might erroneously be acredited with altering
infarct size if it disturbs the kinetics of the CK curve or alters
precordial ST segments (e.g. by effects on heart rate).

3.   HYPOTHESES

Testing the relationship of arrhythmia prevention and limitation of
infarct size requires examination of:

1) whether arrhythmias, particularly ventricular tachycardia and
ventricular fibrillation, increase infarct size.

2) whether prevention of ventricular tachycardia and ventricular
fibrillation limits infarct size.

Investigation of the first hypothesis entails observation of the
natural history of infarction with either direct or indirect assessment of
infarct size. Pre and post arrhythmia assessment of infarct size by
precordial mapping, CK release curves or nuclear imaging is theoretically
possible but is unrealistic in practice as there is insufficient time
prior to the arrhythmia to establish a reliable estimate of extent.
Prognosis provides an indirect assessment of infarct size but is
insensitive and is influenced by many other factors. Pre and post
arrhythmia assessment of prognosis is impossible and comparison of two
infarct populations with and without arrhythmia complications would be

required. The validity of this approach is reduced by the fact that arrhythmias are related to initial infarct size and that both arrhythmias and the reversibility of jeopardised myocardium are time dependent.

Investigation of the second hypothesis is hampered by many of the same problems. In addition, the implication that infarct size restriction by antiarrhythmic therapy might be seen only in those patients destined to develop arrhythmias demands investigation of large patient populations. Moreover, (Figure I) antiarrhythmic therapy, whilst exerting a beneficial effect on one part of the sequence leading from infarction to an alteration in infarct size, might through haemodynamic effects reduce or even reverse the initial useful action. If administered therapy could prove either beneficial or detrimental, the sensitivity of the investigation is reduced.

4.   AVAILABLE EVIDENCE

There is no clinical evidence relating either arrhythmias or the use of administered prophylactic antiarrhythmic therapy to direct estimations of infarct size. The only information concerns the prognosis in patients whose infarction has been complicated by ventricular tachycardia and/or ventricular fibrillation and in patients who have received prophylactic antiarrhythmic therapy.

4.1   Relationship of ventricular tachycardia and ventricular
       fibrillation to prognosis

Several studies have suggested that infarction complicated by primary ventricular fibrillation[9,10,11] (ventricular fibrillation in the absence of shock or cardiac failure) or ventricular tachycardia[12] has an excellent long-term prognosis.

These studies[9,10,11,12] detail the prognosis for survivors of an initial event of ventricular fibrillation or ventricular tachycardia and three[9,10,11] concern the fate of hospital survivors. Ventricular fibrillation and ventricular tachycardia are dangerous arrhythmias and despite appropriate resuscitation both have an appreciable initial mortality[9,10] which is not reflected by these figures. Prevention, if clinically possible, might reduce mortality.

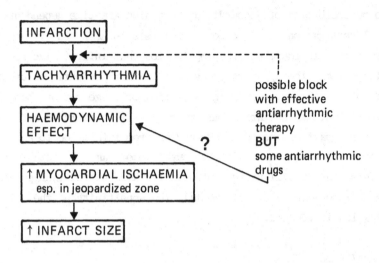

FIGURE I - Relationship of Arrhythmias, Haemodynamic Effects and Infarct
Size

Table I - Prognosis of VF in AMI

	Type of VF	Survival	
		1 year	2 years
Goldberg et al[9]	primary/secondary	80%	
Lie et al[10]	primary	100%(11months)	
Geddes et al[11]	primary	92%	85%
	secondary	58%	30%

In two studies[10,11] in which primary ventricular fibrillation was
clearly separated from secondary and other forms of ventricular
fibrillation, one year survival rates of 92 and 100% and a two year
survival rate of 85% were noted. These figures are little different
from those anticipated for patients with uncomplicated infarction.

Survival rates for patients with secondary ventricular fibrillation (ventricular fibrillation in the presence of shock and/or failure) are much worse[11] and reflect severe underlying myocardial damage and extensive coronary artery disease. Secondary ventricular fibrillation is not considered a preventable phenomenon at this time with the prognosis reflecting extensive anatomic damage rather than the consequences of the electrical instability.

Almost nothing is known of the prognosis of patients whose infarction is complicated by ventricular tachycardia. This in part reflects the lack of a generally agreed definition for ventricular tachycardia. In a single study[12], an excellent long-term prognosis was noted with 94% survival over 19 months. It is unlikely that ventricular tachycardia if defined as three or more consecutive ventricular ectopic complexes at a rate > than 120/minute carries a serious late prognosis as this arrhythmia is detected in up to 50% of patients at some time during the acute phase of infarction[13]. However, the outlook for patients with sustained rapid ventricular tachycardia may be different.

4.2   Prophylactic antiarrhythmic therapy and prognosis

In almost all studies of prophylactic antiarrhythmic therapy in the acute phase of myocardial infarction, the aim has been to reduce arrhythmias, particularly ventricular tachycardia and ventricular fibrillation (Table II). With one exception[21], mortality reduction was not an end point. The mortality figures in Table II are those contained within the original reports. Some reflect mortality during the study period and others mortality for the in-hospital course. The data therefore are not strictly comparable but they provide a basis for examination of the effects of antiarrhythmic therapy on mortality. Many patients were included at a time too late to anticipate that arrhythmia control might have had implications for infarct size but no study excluded patients seen very early after the onset of symptoms.

Prophylactic antiarrhythmic therapy in these investigations has shown an inconsistent effect on the incidence of ventricular fibrillation. In only one study[20] was there a statistically significant reduction. Although ventricular tachycardia appears more reliably reduced, the diagnosis and detection of this event was unreliable in many of the studies. Mortality has not been strikingly influenced by prophylactic antiarrhythmic therapy although a trend for decreased mortality was observed in 9 of the investigations. In two studies, mortality was statistically significantly reduced[18,21], but both were flawed by serious methodological problems and the results have not been confirmed.

Prophylactic non-betablocking antiarrhythmic theraay given to survivors of acute myocardial infarction does not significantly alter mortality[27]. In this context, the antiarrhythmic therapy might have been expected to prevent arrhythmias on reinfarction with the limitation of infarct size being reflected in an improved mortality. The figures do not support this hypothesis

5. CONCLUSIONS

There is little data to indicate that ventricular fibrillation is preventable by the use of non-betablocking antiarrhythmic therapy in acute myocardial infarction. More, though insubstantial, evidence exists for efficacy against ventricular tachycardia. The effect on mortality is neither dramatic nor consistent.

In individual patients the occurrence of a haemodynamically important arrhythmia may be a turning point in their clinical course. It is tempting to postulate that had that arrhythmia been prevented, then the subsequent deterioration, possibly through a mechanism of increased infarct size would not have occurred. Whilst current research cannot deny the possibility of a small effect on infarct size limitation by antiarrhythmic therapy, the data would not support this as a powerful clinical benefit of currently available agents.

Arrhythmias with devastating haemodynamic consequences probably do increase infarct size and even with rapid resuscitation, some ultimately prove fatal. Prophylaxis of these arrhythmias and limitation of myocardial injury is desirable and theoretically feasible but currently available antiarrhythmic agents appear to do neither job well.

Can non-betablocking antiarrhythmic drugs prevent serious ventricular tachyarrhythmias? Will success in using drugs to prevent arrhythmias or limit infarct size be accompanied by frequent adverse effects? Even if infarct size limitation by using prophylactic antiarrhythmic therapy is possible, is the benefit clinically important? Without the answer to these fundamental questions there is at present no evidence upon which to recommend prophylactic antiarrhythmic therapy in an attempt to limit infarct size.

ACKNOWLEDGEMENTS

We should like to acknowledge the invaluable assistance of Mrs. D. Naisby for her help in the preparation of this manuscript.

REFERENCES

1. Braunwald E, Maroko PR: Protection of the Ischemic Myocardium. The Myocardium: Failure and Infarction. HP Publishing Co. Inc., New York, 1974, pp 329.

2. Jurgensen HJ, Frederiksen J, Hansen DA, Sen-Bjergaard OP: Limitation of myocardial infarct size in patients less than 66 years treated with alprenolol. Br Heart J (45):538-8,1981.

3. Adgey AAJ: Pre-hospital coronary care with a mobile unit. In: Collins A ed. Coronary Care in th Community. Croom Helm, London, 1977,pp 97.

4. Reimer KA, Lowe JE, Jennings RB. Effects of the calcium antagonist verapamil on necrosis following temporary coronary artery occlusion in dogs. Circulation (55), 1977, pp 581-587.

5. Nasser FN, Walls JT, Edwards WD, Harrison CE, Dewey JD: Lidocaine induced reduction in size of experimental myocardial infarction. Am J Cardiol (46), 1980, pp 967-75.

6 Schaub RG, Lemole GM, Pinder GC, Black P, Stewart GJ: Effects of lidocaine and epimephrin on myocardial preservation following cardiopulmonary bypass in dog. J Thorac Cardiovasc Surg (74), 1977, pp 571-6.

7. Boudoulas H, Karayannacos PE, Lewis RP, Kakos GS, Kilman JW, Vasko JS: Potential effect of lidocaine on ischemic myocardial injury: experimental and clinical observations. J Surg Res (24), 1978, pp 469-76.

8. Schaub RG, Stewart G, Strong M, Ruotolo R, Lemole G: Reduction of ischemic myocardial damage in the dog by lidocaine infusion. Am J Pathol (87), 1977, pp 399-414.

9. Goldberg R, Szklo M, Kennedy H, Tonascia J: Short and long-term prognosis of myocardial infarction complicated by ventricular fibrillation or cardiac arrest. Circulation (4, supple 2), 1978,pp 89 (abs).

10. Lie KI, Wellens HJJ, Von Capelle FJ, Durrer D: Characteristics and predictability of primary ventricular fibrillation. Eur J Cardiol (1), 1974, pp 379-84.

11. Geddes JS, Adgey AAJ, Pantridge JF: Prognosis after recovery from ventricular fibrillation complicating ischaemic heart disease. Lancet (2), 1969, pp 273-5.

12. De Soyza N, Bennett FA, Murphy ML, Bissett JK, Kane JJ. The relationship of paroxsymal ventricular tachycardia complicating the acute phase of myocardial infarction to long-term survival. Am J Med (64), 1978, pp 377-81.

13. Campbell RWF, Murray A, Julian DG: Ventricular arrhythmias in the first 12 hours of acute myocardial infarction. Natural history study. Br Heart J (46), 1981, pp351-7.

14. Campbell RWF, Hutton I, Elton RA, Goodfellow RM, Taylor E: Prophylaxis of primary ventricular fibrillation with tocainide in acute myocardial infarction. Br Heart J (49), 1983, pp 557-63.

15. Campbell RWF, Bryson LG, Bailey BJ, Murray A, Julian DG: Prophylactic administration of tocainide in acute myocardial infarction. In: Pottage A, Ryden L (eds), Workshop on Tocainide. AB Hassle, Sweden, 1981, pp 201.

16. Campbell RWF, Achuff SC, Pottage A, Murray A, Prescott LF, Julian DG. Mexiletine in the prophylaxis of. ventricular arrhythmias during acute myocardial infarction. J Cardio Pharm (1), 1979, pp 43-52.

17. Lie KI, Liem KL, Louridtz WL, Janse MJ, Willebrands AF, Durrer D. Efficacy of lignocaine in preventing ventricular fibrillation within one hour after a 300mg intramuscular injection. A double-blind randomised study of 300 hospitalised patients with acute myocardial infarction. Am J Cardiol (42), 1978, 486-8.

18. Zainal N, Carmichael DJS, Kidner PH, Gilham AD, Summers GD. Oral disopyramide for the prevention of arrhythmias in patients with acute myocardial infarction admitted to open wards. Lancet (2), 1977, 887-9.

19. Jennings G, Jones MBS, Besterman EMM, Model DG, Turner PP, Kidner PH. Oral disopyramide in prophylaxis of arrhythmias following myocardial infarction. Lancet (1), 1976, pp 51-4.

20. Lie KI, Wellens HJJ, Von Capelle FJ, Durrer D. Lidocaine in the prevention or primary ventricular fibrillation. New Eng J Med (29), 1974, pp 1324-6.

21. Valentine PA, Frew JL, Mashford ML, Sloman JG. Lidocaine in the prevention of sudden death in the pre-hospital phase of acute infarction. New Eng J Med (29), 1974, pp 1327-31.

22. Bleifeld W, Merx W, Heinrich KW, Effert S. Controlled trial of prophylactic treamtnet with lidocaine in acute myocardial infarction. Eur J Clin Pharcol (6), 1973, pp 119-126.

23. O'Brien KP, Taylor PM, Croxson RS. Prophylactic lignocaine in hospitalised patients with acute myocardial infarction. Med J Aust (2), 1973, pp 36-37.

24. Darby S, Bennett SA, Cruickshank JC, Pentecost BL. Trial of combined intramuscular and intravenous lignocaine in proplylaxis of ventricular tachyarrhythmias. Lancet (1), 1972, pp 8179.

25. Pitt A, Lipp J, Anderson ST. Lignocaine given prophylactically to patients with acute myocardial infarction. Lancet (1), 1971, pp 612-5.

26. Bennett MA, Wilner JM, Pentecost BL. Controlled trial of lignocaine in prophylaxis of ventricular arrhythmias complicating myocardial infarction. Lancet (2), 1970, pp 909-11.

27.. May GS, Eberlein KA, Furberg CD, Passamani ER, DeMets DL. Secondary prevention after myocardial infarction: a review of long-term trials. Prog Cardiovasc Dis (24), 1982, pp 331-52.

Table II – Mortality and Antiarrhythmic Effects of Prophylactic Therapy in AMI

Study			Onset of symptoms to inclusion hour	Drug	Route	Arrhythmias	Placebo	Drug	Mortality Placebo	Drug
Campbell et al[14]	1983	(n=559)	<6	Tocainide	iv/o	VF	2%	4%	2%	1%
Campbell et al[15]	1981	(n=68)	<12	Tocainide	o	VF VF/VT	3% 37%	0% 3%	5%	0%
Campbell et al[16]	1979	(n=97)	<12	Mexiletine	o	VF VT	4% 23%	2% 2%	0%	7%
Lie et al[17]	1978	(n=300)	<6	Lidocaine	im	VF	3%	4%	4%	3%
Zainal et al[18]	1977	(n=60)	<36	Disopyramide	o	VF VT	3% 57%	17% 27%	37%	3%
Jennings et al[19]	1976	(n=95)	<48	Disopyramide	o	VF VT	10% 28%	2% 9%	10%	4%
Lie et al[20]	1974	(n=212)	<6	Lidocaine	iv	VF VT	9% 6%	0% 2%	10%	7%
Valentine et al[21]	1974	(n=269)	<12	Lidocaine	im		–	–	7%	2%
Bleifeld et al[22]	1973	(n=99)	<48	Lidocaine	iv	VF VT	4% 10%	0% 7%	8%	5%
O'Brien et al[23]	1973	(n=300)	<24	Lidocaine	iv	VF	3%	5%	3%	7%
Darby et al[24]	1972	(n=203)	<48	Lidocaine	iv/im	VF VT	4% 8%	3% 2%	11%	12%
Pitt et al[25]	1971	(n=222)	<48	Lidocaine	iv	VF	14%	8%	9%	3%
Bennett et al[26]	1970	(n=610)	<48	Lidocaine	iv	VT VI	6% 2%	6% 7%	6%	10%

12

PHARMACEUTICAL INTERVENTIONS TO REDUCE INFARCT SIZE -- STREPTOKINASE

Peter Rentrop. M.D.

Thrombolytic therapy of acute myocardial infarction was first reported by Fletcher et al. in 1959 (1). The authors infused a large dose of Streptokinase intravenously, demonstrating the feasibility of this treatment. In the subsequent years, at least twenty trials were performed in order to assess the efficacy of intravenous thrombolysis in acute myocardial infarction (Table 1). Of the seven trials which showed statistically significant improvement of survival with intravenous Streptokinase therapy, six excluded patients with more than 12 hours of chest pain. The Third European trial demonstrated improved survival in patients with increased risk of mortality, as assessed prospectively on the basis of simple clinical criteria prior to randomization (10).

Whereas Fletcher et al. employed Streptokinase in order to reestablish antegrade flow by dissolving the clot in the acutely obstructed coronary artery, subsequent investigators felt that clot lysis in the main vessel would occur too late to result in any salvage of myocardium (21, 22). It was hypothesized that systemic effects could explain the benefits of thrombolytic therapy seen in some of the trials. The breakdown of fibrinogen results in a reduction of blood viscosity, causing a decrease in afterload (23). In addition, it was suggested that blood flow to the infarct area via collaterals might be improved due to a reduction in viscosity as well as dissolution of microthrombi in collateral vessels (21, 22).

The evolution of coronary angiography into a safe technique, encouraged us to study the coronary artery morphology in patients during the first hours of myocardial infarction (24). In addition, the coronary catheter provided a tool which enabled selective delivery of thrombolytic substance directly to the site of obstruction, resulting in a much higher concentration of the drug at the site of desired action than could be achieved by intravenous infusion (25, 26). Finally, the coronary catheter allowed periodic assessment of the results of thrombolytic therapy during the infusion (25, 26).

Although the technique of intracoronary Streptokinase infusion represents important progress from the investigative point of view, several disadvantages are also obvious. The necessity for acute angiography restricts the application of the procedure to those institutions in which angiographic facilities and trained personnel are available. In addition to the risk of thrombolysis and subsequent anticoagulation, the risk of angiography in the setting of acute infarction must be considered. Therefore any trials, that assess the risk/benefit ratio of intracoronary thrombolytic infusion should have two control groups, ideally: a conventionally treated group in which acute angiography is not performed and a second control group in which acute angiography is performed but thrombolytic therapy is not administered. Such a randomized multicenter trial is being performed at Mount Sinai Hospital, Elmhurst Hospital, and New York University-Bellevue Hospital in New York City. It includes four treatment arms: Group I receives an infusion of intracoronary Streptokinase (2,000 units per minute), Group II receives an infusion of both intracoronary Streptokinase and intracoronary Nitroglycerin (0.01 mg/minute), Group III receives an infusion of intracoronary Nitroglycerin alone; Group IV is treated medically, and not subjected to acute angiography. The

pilot phase of this trial was completed October 31, 1982, after 124 patients had been randomized (27).

Acute recanalization rates were: Group I- 12/19; Group II- 19/23; Group III- 1/18. While the differences between Groups I and II did not achieve statistical significance, both groups showed significantly higher recanalization rates than Group III (27). In the literature, acute recanalization rates between 60-90% have been reported (28, 29).

Mortality data in various small randomized trials have been conflicting (27, 30). Pooling the data from eight randomized trials, Furberg calculated a mortality of 11% in Streptokinase treated patients (n= 42/382) and of 12.4% in the control group (n= 45/364) (31). In view of this small difference, it may be useful to try to

identify subgroups of patients in whom the beneficial effects of
thrombolytic therapy can be expected to be more marked.

Since the ejection fraction in the acute stage of infarction correlates
well with prognosis (32), we have analysed change of ejection fraction
in 125 patients who had contrast ventriculography prior to
Streptokinase infusion and a repeat study prior to hospital discharge
(33). Improvement of ejection fraction was found to correlate with
incomplete obstruction of the infarct vessel at the time of
preintervention angiography, with the presence of angiographically
demonstrable collaterals to the infarct area and with recanalization of
complete coronary obstruction. Based on the data of patients in whom
recanalization of complete obstruction was achieved, a model was
developed relating extent of ejection fraction improvement to
preintervention ejection fraction and duration of infarct pain prior to
hospital admission. The largest increase of ejection fraction occurred
when preintervention ejection fraction was low and the patient was
treated immediately after the onset of infarct symptoms. The increase
of ejection fraction became small at about three hours after the onset
of pain. However, these narrow time constraints may not apply in
patients with incomplete coronary obstruction or well-developed
collaterals.

Intracoronary Streptokinase infusion is associated with several
problems in patient management. First, hemodynamically unstable
patients may not tolerate dye injection; further, they may be unable to
maintain a recumbent position on the catheterization table. These

factors, as well as the potential need for resuscitative efforts, may interfere with the efficacy of this procedure. We have found intraaortic balloon counterpulsation during the intervention to be useful in controlling these problems.

Second, reperfusion arrhythmias can be dangerous in patients with severely depressed left ventricular function. In addition, we have seen severe transient deterioration of left ventricular function after reperfusion. These problems are also best handled by early intraaortic balloon counterpulsation in patients with severely depressed left ventricular function.

Third, reocclusion after successful recanalization is associated with a high risk of fatal reinfarction (34), necessitating anticoagulation with Heparin for at least 4 days following reperfusion

Fourth, there is a risk of significant bleeding due to thrombolytic therapy and subsequent anticoagulation (34), necessitating exclusion of all patients susceptible to life threatening bleeding complications.

Fifth, the rate of secondary interventions, such as intraaortic balloon counterpulsation, angioplasty and coronary artery bypass surgery, tends to be higher in patients treated with intracoronary Streptokinase infusion. The risk of these interventions has to be considered when assessing the efficacy of intracoronary thrombolytic therapy.

TABLE 1:

MORTALITY IN INTRAVENOUS THROMBOLYTIC THERAPY TRIALS

TRIAL	YEAR PUBLISHED	HOURS*	MORTALITY SK/CONTROL (%)	P
FIRST GERMAN- SWISS[2]	(1966)	12	14.1/21.7	<0.05
ITALIAN[3]	(1971)	12	11.6/11.4	NS
SECOND GERMAN- SWISS[4]	(1973)	12	14.5/26.0	<0.03
FRANKFURT PILOT[5]	(1973)	12	18.7/21.1	NS
FRANFURT (RANDOMIZED)[5]	(1973)	12	12.8/27.6	<0.01
EUROPEAN COLLABORATIVE[6] (UK)	(1975)	12	23.3/22.2	NS
TOURS[7]	(1975)	12	2/13	<0.025
AUSTRIAN[8]	(1976)	12	10.5/17.3	<0.01
GRAZ[9]	(1976)	12	28/11	NS
THIRD EUROPEAN[10]	(1979)	12	15.6/30.6	<0.01
PLASMIN -UK [11]	(1965)	48	14/17	NS
FIRST EUROPEAN[12]	(1969)	72	16.7/17.8	NS
PLASMIN -SK[13]	(1969)	24	26/34	-
FINNISH[14]	(1971)	72	10/8.2	NS
SECOND EUROPEAN[15]	(1971)	24	18.5/26.3	<0.025
DANISH[16]	(1972)	24	23.1/29.4	NS
AUSTRALIAN[17]	(1973)	24	10.9/12.8	NS
DANISH (UK)[18]	(1973)	24	14.3/21.4	-
NHLI PILOT[19]	(1974)	24	---	-
UNITED KINGDOM[20]	(1976)	24	14.2/15.0	NS

HOURS* = Maximum duration of infarct pain prior to entry into the trial.

1. Fletcher AP, Sherry S, Alkjaersig N, et al: The maintenance of a sustained thrombolytic state in man II. Clinical observations on patients with myocardial infarciton and other thrombo-embolic disorder. J Clin Invest 38:1111, 1959.

2. Schmutzler R, Heckner F, Koertge P, et al: Zur thrombolytischen Therapie des frischen Herzinfarktes. I Einfuehrung, Behandlungsplaene. Allgemeine klinische Ergebnisse. Dtsch Med Wochenschr 91:581, 1966.

3. Dioguardi N, Mannucci PM, Lotto A, et al: Controlled trial of streptokinase and heparin in acute myocardial infarction. Lancet 2:891, 1971.

4. Schmutzler R, Fritze E, Gebauer D, et al: Fibrinolytic therapy in acute myocardial infarction, Thromb Diath Haemorrh (Suppl)47:211, 1971.

5. Breddin K, Ehrly HM, Fechler L, et al: Die Kurzzeitfibrinolyse beim akuten Myocardinfarkt. Dtsch Med Wochenschr 98:861, 1973.

6. European Collaborative Study: Controlled trial of urokinase in myocardial infarction. Lancet 2:624, 1975.

7. Brochier M, Raynaud R, Planiol T, et al: Le traitement par l'urokinase des infarctus du myocarde et syndromes de menace. Etude randomisee de 120 cas. Arch Mal Coeur 68:563, 1975.

8. Haider M, Ambrosch L, Groll-Knapp E, et al: Ergebnisse der Oestereichischen Herzinfarkstudie, in Sailer S (ed): Die Fibrinolyse-Behandlung des akuten Myokard-Infarktes. Wien, Verlag Brueder Hollinek, 45, 1976.

9. Klein W, Pavek P, Brandt D, et al: Resultate einer Doppelblindstudie beim Myokardinfarkt, in Sailer S(ed): Die Fibrinolyse-Behandlung des akuten Myokard-Infarktes. Wien, Verlag Brueder Hollinek, 65, 1976.

10. European Cooperative Study Group for Streptokinase Treatment in Acute Myocardial Infarction. Streptokinase in acute myocardial infarction. N Engl J Med. 301:797, 1979.

11. Lippschutz EJ, Ambrus JL, Ambrus CM, et al: Controlled study on the treatment of coronary occlusion with urokinase-activated human plasmin. Am J Cardiol 16:93, 1965.

12. Amery A, Roeber G, Vermeulen HJ, et al: Single-blind randomised multicentre trial comparing heparin and streptokinase treatment in recent myocardial infarction. Acta Med Scand 187 (Suppl 505):5, 1969.

13. Richter IH, Epstein S, Cliffton E: An evaluation of fibrinolysis therapy in acute myocardial infarction. Angiology 20:95, 1969.

14. Heikinheimo R, Ahrenberg P, Honkapohja H, et al: Fibrinolytic treatment in myocardial infarction. Acta Med Scand 189:7, 1971.

15. European Working Party: Streptokinase in recent myocardial infarction: A controlled multicentre trial. Br Med J 3:325, 1971.

16. Gormsen J: Biochemical evaluation of standard treatment with streptokinase in acute myocardial infarction. Acta Med Scand 191:77, 1972.

17. Bett JHN, Biggs JC, Castaldi PA, et al: Australian multicentre trial of streptokinase in acute myocardial infarction. Lancet 1:57, 1973.

18. Gormsen J, Tidstrom B, Feddersen C, et al: Biochemical evaluation of low dose of urokinase in acute myocardial infarction. A double blind study. Acta Med Scand 194:191, 1973.

19. Ness PM, Simon TL, Cole C, et al: A pilot study of streptokinase study in acute myocardial infarction: observations on complications and relation to trial design. Am Heart J 88:705,1974.

20. Aber CP, Bass NM, Berry CL, et al: Streptokinase in acute myocardial infarction: A controlled multicentre study in the United Kingdom. Br Med 12:1100, 1976.

21. Bouvier CA, Ruegsegger P, Nydick I: Etude histologique de l'effet d'enzymes fibrinolytiques sur l'evolution d'un infarctus experimental chez le chien. Helvetica Med Acta, 516:656, 1960.

22. Ruegsegger P, Nydick I, Abarquez R: Effect of fibrinolytic (Plasmin) therapy on the physiopathology of myocardial infarction. Amer J Cardiol, 519, 1960.

23. Neuhof H, Hey D, Glaser E, et al: Hemodynamic reactions induced by streptokinase therapy in patients with acute myocardial infarction. Eur J Intensiv. Care Med., 1:27, 1975.

24. Rentrop P, Blanke H, Karsch KR: Koronarmorphologie und linksventrikulaere Pumpfunktion im akuten Infarkstadium und ihre Aenderung im chronischen Stadium. Z. Kardiol. 68:335, 1979.

25. Rentrop P, Blanke H, Karsch KR, et. al: Acute myocardial infarction: Intracoronary application of nitroglycerin and streptokinase in combination with transluminal recanalization. Clin. Cardiol. 2:354, 1979.

26. Rentrop P, Blanke H, Karsch KR, et. al: Selective intracoronary thrombolysis in acute myocardial infarction and unstable angina pectoris. Circulation 63:307, 1981.

27. Rentrop P, Feit F, Schneider R, et. al: Mt. Sinai- New York University randomized reperfusion trial: Pilot phase. J Amer Col. Cardiol., In Press.

28. Khaja F, Walton Jr. J, Brymer J, et al.: Intracoronary fibrinolytic therapy in acute myocardial infarction. N Eng J Med, 303:22, 1983.

29. Saltups A, Boxall J, Ho B, et. al: Intracoronary vs. intravenous streptokinase in acute myocardial infarction. Circulation 68:III-119, 1983.

30. Kennedy J, Ritchie J, Davis K, et al.: The western washington streptokinase in acute myocardial infarction randomized trial. Circulation, 68:III-23, 1983.

31. Furberg C: Clinical Value of Intracoronary Streptokinase. Am J Cardiol, In Press.

32. Shah PK, Pichler M, Berman DS, et. al.: Left ventricular ejection fraction determined by radionuclide ventriculography in early stages of first transmural infarction. Relation to short-term prognosis. Am J Cardiol 45:542, 1980.

33. Rentrop P, Smith H, Painter L, Holt J: Changes in left ventricular ejection fraction after intracoronary thrombolytic therapy. Results of the Registry of the European Society of Cardiology. Circulation, 68:I-55, 1983.

34. Merx W, Doerr R, Rentrop P, et. al: Intracoronary infusion of streptokinase in acute myocardial infarction. Postacute management and hospital course in 204 patients. Am Heart J 102:1181, 1981.

13

STREPTOKINASE IN ACUTE MYOCARDIAL INFARCTION

SIDNEY GOLDSTEIN, M.D., AND FAREED KHAJA, M.D.

It is axiomatic that reperfusion of an occluded coronary artery, before irreversible damage has occurred, will improve function of the jeopardized myocardial tissue. Having thus accepted reperfusion as an important principal in the treatment of myocardial infarction, we would like to raise questions in regard to the methodology, effectiveness, and appropriateness of thrombolytic therapy currently performed using streptokinase. We will challenge the role of thrombosis as a cause of acute myocardial infarction; discuss the time frame in which thrombolysis must occur in order to restore both flow and function; investigate what we currently know about the effect of reperfusion on restoring ventricular function and improved mortality; and consider both the logistics and the risk of the current clinical practice of streptokinase therapy.

The importance of thrombosis in the pathogenesis of acute myocardial infarction has been reemphasized in the recent literature. The timing at which the thrombosis occurs is particularly important in patients with transmural myocardial infarction with defined Q waves and enzyme elevation. Thrombosis is present in greater than 80% of patients examined within the first six hours of the onset of symptoms[1]. Superficially, this appears to be an obvious association between thrombosis and infarction. In many things, however, what is obvious is not always correct. As one pursues the ischemic event closer to its onset in patients, for instance, who die suddenly[2] or with unstable angina[3], the occurrence of thrombosis

is rare. Similarly, as one moves farther in time from the development
of symptoms, thrombosis becomes a less frequent occurrence. These observations have important implications at both ends of the temporal spectrum.
It appears that the thrombosis is most important at a time when acute
necrosis is in progress, suggesting perhaps that it is a concurrent or
even a secondary event rather than the primary cause of infarction.
Therefore, thrombolysis may be advocated at a time when the dye has
already been cast and the extent of myocardial damage already been determined.
It is possible that thrombosis may lead to propagation of clots throughout
the distal coronary vascular tree supplied by the occluded artery, thereby,
interfering with collateral blood in support of peripheral infarct zones.
Thrombolytic therapy, therefore, may be more important in the lysis of
smaller clots in the peripheral ramifications of the occluded coronary
vessel. We have observed, on occasion, better collateral visualization
after reperfusion with intracoronary streptokinase than with spontaneous
reperfusion in the setting of post-infarction angina. This hypothesis,
however, is untested.

The measurement of the effectiveness of reperfusion remains a major
issue in current clinical research and hinges on our inability to accurately
measure infarct size. Although animal models have demonstrated that there
is improved segmental contraction with reperfusion within three hours of
occlusion[4], there is little evidence to suggest that reperfusion beyond
three hours is effective. In fact, most data would suggest that reperfusion
established after three hours is ineffective in improving myocardial function. At any time, reperfusion after one hour fails to improve global
left ventricular function in animals   [4]. It has been suggested that
the time limit for thrombolysis in man may be longer than in animals because
of the development of collaterals in man with long-standing coronary heart

reperfusion does not indicate viability of the reperfused myocardial tissue[9]. Thus, clinical observations in post myocardial infarction patients would hinge on the fact that improved survivorship is closely linked to improved global left ventricular ejection rather than segmental ejection measurements. The importance of improvement in segmental ejection remains to be established.

The knowledge about the effect of streptokinase therapy on mortality is limited. Preliminary studies by Kennedy et al.[10] suggest that there is improvement in mortality in their randomized study. That study, however, unfortunately exhibited a disproportionate number of high risk patients in the placebo population but did result in a statistical improvement in mortality in streptokinase therapy group. Intravenous studies in a European cooperative trial[11] suggested that there was improvement in survivorship, although there was a substantial degree of morbidity associated with the prolonged administration of IV streptokinase.

The logistics of streptokinase therapy also pose major problems. Early administration is unquestionably important. The need for early administration almost excludes the use of intracoronary injection. Using a cutoff period of six hours, less than 20% of the patients entering our coronary care unit with acute myocardial infarction were candidates for intracoronary injection[5]. It is possible that intravenous injection can be started in less than three hours of infarction, but based upon our six-hour experience, it will be applicable to an even smaller number of patients. Advocates of streptokinase therapy have suggested that the drug should be administered before the development of Q waves and ST segment elevation indicative of ischemia. Yet, in this area, as noted previously, there is a significant question as to whether or not thrombosis plays a role at that time.

Weighed against the dubious success of early administration are the risks of this therapy. Khaja et al.[5] noted a 4% mortality rate,

disease. In both our own study[5] and that of Leiboff et al.[6], the presence

of collaterals was not beneficial to the survival of myocardial tissue.

Furthermore, only 50% of patients with acute infarction have any angio-

graphically visible collaterals to jeopardized zone. It is also important

to emphasize that the animal model in which most studies have been carried

out is particularly rich in collaterals, which develop within minutes of

coronary occlusion. The canine model is, therefore, an optimistic approxi-

mation of the effect of reperfusion relative to collateral pathways.

Randomized studies indicate there is no salutory effect on global

ejection fraction following reperfusion. The study by Khaja et al.[5]

indicates there is no benefit on global or regional ejection fraction in

streptokinase-treated patients compared to control patients. In a recent

uncontrolled study in man, however, it appears that there is improvement

in segmental contractions in areas of reperfusion with no improvement in

total ejection fraction[7]. Much has been made of the fact that total

ejection fraction should not be used as a measurement of improvement of

left ventricular function. Those who argue for this suggest that since

coronary artery disease is a focal disease, one should look at localized

areas of improvement of ejection fraction rather than measuring global

ejection fraction. Nevertheless, the major index of prognosis following

acute myocardial infarction is not regional but global ejection fraction[8].

Even if regional wall motion improves in the jeopardized myocardium following

reperfusion, its contribution to global ejection fraction has been negligible.

Therefore, we can presume that its effect on improved prognosis following

infarction will be negligible. Measurement of the salvaged myocardium is

fraught with significant limitations, both in methodology between inter-

observer and intraobserver differences. Although reperfusion has been

demonstrated using radioisotope thallium[201], recent studies indicate this

associated with cardiac catheterization and streptokinase therapy. Bolus
rather than prolonged intravenous administration of the drug may result
in fewer adverse reactions. If this technique were extended to larger
populations with inadequate monitoring, the potential for morbidity and
mortality could outweigh the possible benefits. Development of gastro-
intestinal and intracranial bleeding are not to be minimized. We have
observed both of these phenomenon during the use of high dose intravenous
streptokinase therapy.

Before we accept routine clinical use of streptokinase in the treatment of acute myocardial infarction, methodologic problems to assess infarct
size and salvage of jeopardized myocardium must be addressed and extended
to the cellular metabolic studies. If thrombosis does occur as a prelude
to acute myocardial infarction, the marker and timing for it in relation
to pain and EKG changes needs to be identified. Longterm prospective
randomized trials are clearly warranted in order to identify the specific
patients with coronary heart disease who will benefit from this therapy.

REFERENCES

1. DeWood MA, Spores J, Notske R, Mouser LT, Burroughs R, Golden MS,
    Lang HT: Prevalence of total coronary occlusion during the early
    hours of transmural myocardial infarction. N Engl J Med 303:897,
    1980.
2. Roberts WC, Buja LM: The frequency and significance of coronary
    arterial thrombi and other observations in fatal acute myocardial
    infarction. A study of 107 necropsy patients. Am J Med 52:425,
    1972.
3. Rentrop P, Blanke H, Karsch KR, Kaiser H, Kostering H, Leitz K:
    Selective intracoronary thrombolysis in acute myocardial infarction
    and unstable angina pectoris. Circulation 63:307, 1981.
4. Lavallee M, Cox D, Patrick TA, Vatner SF: Salvage of myocardial
    function by coronary artery reperfusion 1, 2, and 3 hours after
    occlusion in conscious dogs. Circ Res 53:235, 1983.
5. Khaja F, Walton JA, Brymer JF, Lo E, Osterberger L, O'Neill WW,
    Colfer HT, Weiss R, Lee T, Kurian T, Goldberg AD, Pitt B, Goldstein S:
    Intracoronary fibrinolytic therapy in acute myocardial infarction:
    Report of a prospective randomized trial. N Engl J Med 308:1305,
    1983.

6. Leiboff RH, Katz RJ, Wasserman AG, Bren GB, Schwartz H, Varghese PJ, Ross AM: A randomized angiographically controlled trial of intracoronary streptokinase in acute myocardial infarction. Submitted for publication.

7. Stack RS, Phillips HR III, Grierson DS, Behar VS, Kong Y, Peter RH, Swain JL, Greenfield JC Jr: Functional improvement of jeopardized myocardium following intracoronary streptokinase infusion in acute myocardial infarction. J Clin Invest 72:84, 1983.

8. The Multicenter Postinfarction Research Group: Risk stratification and survival after myocardial infarction. N Engl J Med 309:331, 1983.

9. Melin JA, Becker LC, Bulkley BH: Differences in thallium-201 uptake in reperfused and nonreperfused myocardial infarction. Circ Res 53:414, 1983.

10. Principal Investigators and Their Associates: The western Washington intracoronary streptokinase in acute myocardial infarction randomized trial: Analysis of early mortality. Submitted for publication.

11. European Cooperative Study Group for Streptokinase Treatment in Acute Myocardial Infarction: Streptokinase in acute myocardial infarction. N Engl J Med 301:797, 1979.

14

VASODILATORS IN ACUTE MYOCARDIAL INFARCTION

JAY N. COHN

The use of vasodilators in the treatment of acute
myocardial infarction is rooted in observations demonstrating
that these drugs acutely improve left ventricular performance,
which is significantly impaired in a majority of patients
with acute myocardial infarction (1). Early studies with
intravenous infusion of nitroprusside (2) or with sublingual
or intravenous administration of nitroglycerin (3,4)
demonstrated that these drugs produce a sharp reduction in
left ventricular filling pressure often associated with an
increase in cardiac output. Thus the depressed left
ventricular function curve was shifted by these agents
upward and to the left reflecting improved global performance
of the left ventricle.

Although improving the function of the left ventricle
might be beneficial in patients with acute myocardial
infarction, particularly when the infarction is accompanied
by signs of severe pump failure, a decision about therapeutic
efficacy of such an intervention must be based on more
extensive observations. Consideration must be given to the
effect of the intervention on myocardial ischemia, the
influence on arrhythmias which may be life threatening, the
effect on eventual infarct size, and most importantly the
effect on the mortality in acute myocardial infarction. An
understanding of all of these possible effects of nitroprusside,
nitroglycerin or other vasodilators is necessary before
rational advice can be offered about the appropriateness
of use of these agents in the setting of acute myocardial
infarction.

Several lines of evidence suggest that these agents may under appropriate circumstances relieve myocardial ischemia. Although nitroglycerin has served as the standard agent for relieving anginal attacks, it has long been taught that this drug should not be administered in the presence of acute myocardial infarction. This admonition apparently is related to the possible hypotensive effect of nitroglycerin in certain susceptible individuals. In practice, however, cautious administration of nitroglycerin, particularly in an intravenous form that allows for moment-to-moment titration, produces only a modest fall in arterial pressure with a prominent reduction in the left ventricular filling pressure and frequently with a reduction in ST segment elevation in leads reflecting myocardial injury (4,5). Furthermore, acute relief of the ischemic chest pain accompanying acute myocardial infarction has been reported in response to both nitroglycerin and sodium nitroprusside (6).

Studies of the effect of either nitroprusside or nitroglycerin on serum creatine kinase enzyme release has been reported in at least two large scale studies of acute myocardial infarction (7,8). In both instances a 48 hour infusion of nitroglycerin or nitroprusside resulted in a significant reduction of total serum CK or CK-MB release consistent with a reduction of myocardial infarct size. However, a variety of factors, including alterations in myocardial perfusion, in the enzyme distribution volume or in the enzyme disappearance rate also could contribute to changes in serum enzyme activity. Therefore, although these data are consistent with a reduction in infarct size by the vasodilators, enzyme data alone cannot be used to conclude that infarct size was reduced.

In order to evaluate the benefit: risk ratio of adminis-tration of sodium nitroprusside to patients with acute myocardial infarction a VA cooperative study was initiated in 1975 to evaluate the effect on mortality of a 48 hour infusion of sodium nitroprusside administered to a group of

patients with acute myocardial infarction complicated by
elevated left ventricular filling pressure. Results of the
effects of this intervention on mortality rate have already
been published (8). The study group consisted of 812
patients who had a pulmonary wedge pressure of greater than
12 mmHg within the first 24 hours after their chest pain of
acute myocardial infarction. The study group represented
less than 25% of the patients screened for participation in
the study in the coronary care units of 11 Veterans
Administration Hospitals. The other patients were excluded
for a number of reasons, the most common being that pulmonary
wedge pressure was less than 12 mmHg, that the findings did
not corroborate the diagnosis of acute myocardial infarction,
or that the chest pain was more than 24 hours prior to the
time of screening for randomization into the study. Patients
with shock were excluded from participation. Randomized
patients were assigned double-blind to receive either
sodium nitroprusside or placebo intravenously for 48 hours
in a dose titrated to produce a 40% reduction in the
control pulmonary wedge pressure or to produce a maximum
depression of arterial pressure or to reach a maximum infusion
rate which represented 200 mcg/min of nitroprusside or a
comparable rate of placebo infusion.

Since 405 of the patients were randomized to a placebo
infusion and were therefore treated with conventional
therapy for acute myocardial infarction, this experience
provided rich data related to the current experience with
acute myocardial infarction. In this placebo group the 13
week mortality from acute myocardial infarction was
linearly related to the control pulmonary wedge pressure
and was strikingly and independently related to age.
Indeed, a logistic regression model incorporating all
available clinical and hemodynamic data revealed that
pulmonary wedge pressure and age were the most powerful
predictors of mortality and that the only additional
variables that affected the prediction were a history of
congestive heart failure, the presence of left bundle

branch block and lateral wall involvement by ECG criteria. Using this regression model it was possible to identify a group with predicted survival greater than 90% (actual survival 94%) and another group with predicted survival less than 30% (actual survival 8%). These data remind us of the heterogeneity of risk in patients who sustain an acute myocardial infarction and demonstrate that this risk can be remarkably well predicted simply by measuring the pulmonary wedge pressure and knowing the age. Therefore, clinical trials that do not assess and stratify for these two variables may run the risk of imbalance that could profoundly affect mortality.

During infusion of nitroprusside in this study the pulmonary wedge pressure fell promptly and remained at this level for the ensuing 48 hours. Arterial pressure also showed a sharp decline at the onset of infusion of nitroprusside and remained at this low level throughout the 48 hours of infusion. In the placebo group there was a trend for a gradual reduction in both arterial pressure and pulmonary wedge pressure so that by 40 hours the pressures in the two groups were indistinguishable. Heart rate changes in the nitroprusside group were not significantly different than the heart rate changes in the placebo group.

The effect on mortality was a surprise. Overall mortality was not influenced and was similar in both the placebo and nitroprusside-treated groups. However, when response to therapy was studied separately in those patients who were begun on the infusion within the first 9 hours after the onset of their myocardial infarction compared to those who were begun on therapy greater than 9 hours after the onset of their myocardial infarction, a striking difference was observed. In the early-treated patients nitroprusside appeared to have an adverse effect on 13 week mortality, particularly when the control pulmonary wedge pressure was only slightly or moderately increased. In patients in whom wedge pressure was greater than 22 mmHg this adverse effect of nitroprusside disappeared. In contrast, in the subgroup

treated with nitroprusside more than 9 hours after the
onset of their myocardial infarction the nitroprusside
infusion appeared to have a favorable effect on mortality
regardless of the degree of elevation of pulmonary wedge
pressure. This striking difference between the early-
treated and late-treated groups may be less cryptic than it
seems when one recognizes that the two patient populations
may be strikingly different. Since pulmonary wedge
pressure fell spontaneously in the placebo patient group it
would be anticipated that the longer the interval between
the onset of the myocardial infarction and the time of the
study, the more likely would the pulmonary wedge pressure
have fallen below 12 mmHg which would make the patient
ineligible for study. Consequently, those patients who
were randomized and begun on therapy more than 9 hours
after onset of the event probably represented a more
seriously ill patient population with pump failure that had
not adequately been corrected by spontaneous reduction of
the wedge pressure over the first few hours in the hospital.
Furthermore these data suggest that modest elevations of
pulmonary wedge pressure in the first few hours after a
myocardial infarction may in many instances be viewed as a
transient phenomenon that will spontaneously resolve during
the first day in the hospital.

Another controlled trial of sodium nitroprusside in
patients with acute mycardial infarction has demonstrated a
reduction of mortality in the treated group, particularly
in patients begun on the therapy early (9). The reason for
the discrepancy between this smaller study carried out in
the Netherlands and the larger VA cooperative study is not
entirely clear, but one possibility relates to the strikingly
different mortality experience in the two studies. In the
Netherlands study approximately one-half of the deaths were
due to myocardial rupture which was a rare phenomenon in
the VA cooperative study. Since rupture may be directly
related to left ventricular wall stresses which are directly
related to the arterial pressure it is not surprising that a

patient population unusually prone to myocardial rupture might exhibit a beneficial effect of blood pressure lowering by use of sodium nitroprusside. In addition, the Netherlands study did not include hemodynamic monitoring, and an imbalance of pulmonary wedge pressure between the two groups could explain the mortality difference. Furthermore, the differences in mortality between the two groups was small and appeared to be diminishing with a longer period of observation.

Recent studies reported from the Johns Hopkins University have reported a possible beneficial effect of a 48 hour infusion of nitroglycerin in patients with acute myocardial infarction (10). This study also was small in size and did not demonstrate a difference in mortality in the placebo and nitroglycerin treated groups. However, radioactive ejection fractions performed in the acute phase and during the recovery phase of acute myocardial infarction demonstrated a trend for the ejection fraction to increase in patients treated with nitroglycerin, particularly when the nitroglycerin infusion was initiated early after the onset of myocardial infarction, compared to the placebo group that exhibited no such increase in ejection fraction.

Taken together these observations may be used to place in perspective the use of vasodilators in acute myocardial infarction. It is clear that vasodilators of all types may improve left ventricular performance and in some patients relieve myocardial ischemia by virtue of a systemic or coronary vascular effect. It is also clear that prognosis in myocardial infarction is good when the left ventricular filling pressure is normal or only slightly elevated. Therefore, efficacy of treatment on mortality in this patient population will be exceedingly difficult to demonstrate. The results of the nitroprusside controlled trial suggest that infusion of this drug in the early stages of an uncomplicated myocardial infarction could have a deleterious effect on prognosis but that administration of this drug may be beneficial when given to patients whose

myocardial infarction is complicated by heart failure that
persists for more than 9 hours.

On the basis of these data we would suggest the
following guidelines for vasodilator therapy at the present
time: 1) In patients with uncomplicated myocardial infarction
and an assumed or measured normal left ventricular filling
pressure there is no indication for administration of vasodilator
drugs. 2) In myocardial infarction complicated by persistant
pain suggesting continuing ischemia the administration of
nitroglycerin intraveneously appears to be appropriate.
3) In myocardial infarction complicated by an asymptomatic
elevation of left ventricular filling pressure in the first
8 hours after acute myocardial infarction the physician may
wait for spontaneous fall of this elevated filling pressure
or might be inclined to use nitroglycerin which must be
adminstered without evidence that it will have a favorable
effect on the course. A diuretic agent often is used in
these patients and was administered to many of the patients
in the VA cooperative study. 4) In patients with myocardial
infarction and an elevated left ventricular filling pressure
which has persisted for at least 9 hours after myocardial
infarction, treatment with nitroprusside appears to be
appropriate. 5) In myocardial infarction with a low output
pump failure state either early or late in the course of
acute myocardial infarction, administration of nitroprusside
often with other agents is physiologically rational and
appears to be effective.

REFERENCES

1. Hamosh P, Cohn JN: Left ventricular function in acute
   myocardial infarction. J Clin Invest (50):523-533,
   1971.
2. Franciosa JA, Guiha NH, Limas CJ, Rodriguera E, Cohn JN:
   Improved left ventricular function during nitroprusside
   infusion in acute myocardial infarction. Lancet (1):
   650-654, 1972.
3. Gold HK, Leinbach RC, Sanders CS: Use of sublingual
   nitroglycerin in congestive failure following acute
   myocardial infarction. Circulation (46):839-845, 1973.

4. Flaherty JT, Reid PR, Kelly DT, Taylor DR, Weisfeldt ML, Pitt B: Intravenous nitroglycerin in acute myocardial infarction. Circulation (51):132-139, 1975.

5. Epstein SE, Kent KM, Goldstein RE, Borer J, Redwood D: Reduction of ischemic injury by nitroglycerin during acute myocardial infarction. N Engl J Med (292):29-35, 1975.

6. Mukherjee D, Feldman MS, Helfant RH: Nitroprusside therapy: treatment of hypertensive patients with recurrent resting chest pain, ST-segment elevation, and ventricular arrhythmias. JAMA (235):2406-2409, 1976.

7. Bussmann W-D, Passek D, Seidel W, Kaltenbach M: Reduction of CK and CK-MB Indexes of infarct size by intravenous nitroglycerin. Circulation (63):615-622, 1981.

8. Cohn JN, Franciosa JA, Francis GS, Archibald D, Tristani F, Fletcher R, Montero A, Cintron G, Clarke J, Hager D, Saunders R, Cobb F, Smith R, Loeb H, Settle H: Effect of short-term infusion of sodium nitroprusside on mortality rate in acute myocardial infarction complicated by left ventricular failure. New Engl J Med (306):1129-1135, 1982.

9. Durrer JD, Lie KI, van Capelle FJL, Durrer D: Effect of sodium nitroprusside on mortality in acute myocardial infarction. New Engl J Med (306):1121-1128, 1982.

10. Flaherty JT, Becker LC, Bulkley BH, Weiss JL, Gerstenblith G, Kallman CH, Silverman KJ, Wei JY, Pitt B, Weisfeldt ML: A randomized prospective trial of intravenous nitroglycerin in patients with acute myocardial infarction. Circulation (68):576-588, 1983.

15

PANEL ON PHARMACEUTICAL INTERVENTIONS TO REDUCE INFARCT SIZE

Moderator: Dr. Jay Cohn

Dr. Ruberio: We were interested in of lidocaine for a long time. From
the 13 clinical trials, 11 were negative and 2 were positive and we are
confused with that. We decided to study the effects of lidocaine after
myocardial infarction, after coronary ligation in dogs, and I would like to
quickly share with you what we found. We showed that the antiarrhythmic
effect of lidocaine after coronary artery occlusion has not to do only with
the blood level but with the myocardial lidocaine concentration. If we
separate the dogs that responded from the dogs that did not respond, the
blood levels were exactly the same, but the myocardial lidocaine level was
different. Since lidocaine has membrane stabilizing effects and since it
is demonstrated that lidocaine is a vasodilator by microsphere technique,
we decided to check it in reduction of infarct size. We found that lidocaine reduced infarct size by 20% and it had nothing to do with the antiarrhythmic effect. In those animals the mortality wasn't different and
they didn't have arrhythmias in the first 6 hours in which they were
evaluated. There is a protective effect which has nothing to do with the
antiarrhythmic effect and if we can give lidocaine to patients with acute
myocardial infarction without causing toxicity, I think we should do that
instead of waiting for statistical significance. We all know that the only
drugs at this moment that have effected mortality are the beta blockers. If
we have to wait for statistical significance, I think we are going to miss
the boat.

Dr. Cohn :   Now there is a strong statement. I knew there was a reason
why we put this discussion under limitation of infarct size. Any comments?

Dr. Harrison: First, I don't want to start another controversy, but extrapolating from animal models of infarct size to human studies is perilous at
best in my view at this point in time. I am not trying to make that as the
reason for the prophylactic administration of lidocaine. I think that when

you have VF or when you have tachyarrhythmias and even if you have proper rescusitation you are going to lose a certain number of myocardial cells and if you can prevent that safely I would like to believe that that reduces infarct size.

Dr. Campbell: I warmed to what you were saying because I thought you were going to come down on my side on the end of it, but I alluded to your work in fact. I am aware of these animal effects of lidocaine, but I would agree with Don, that I don't think you can extrapolate these to man. I share your concern about the 13 published studies and there are many more in fact. If that most important study by Lie were un-impeachable in all its respects, its conduct, its size, etc., then perhaps I would accept the data more gladly. I think there are so many problems with that and there are so many who use prophylactic lidocaine therapy with that as the pivotal reason for doing so, I think that is wrong. I would like to see that repeated. That is why I would say for the moment, I would hold my hand on prophylactic therapy. Once you do it, it is very difficult to go back on.

Dr. Temple: The logical sequence that you used Don to advocate prophy-laxis was that there was life-table evidence that having an arrhythmia that needs resuscitation was bad for you because those don't survive as well and that you can prevent those arrhythmias as shown by the Lie study. As I am sure you realize, the sequence is not air tight. What that showed was that people who are of a nature and condition, such as to develop an arrhythmia that needs resuscitation have a worse prognosis, it really doesn't prove that the arrhythmia itself was the cause of that. Obviously that is a problem there. Do I take it you were each talking about the same study that pooled several lidocaine prophylaxis studies?

Dr. Harrison: There were several studies.

Dr. Temple: One of the things that is popular now is to pool a lot of studies and reach a conclusion that seems stronger than the components and this is obviously another example of that. The pooled data is primarily the effect of the Lie study and nothing but the Lie study when you look at the total difference.

Dr. Harrison: But it is the best control. It is the one where they had
plasma levels where they used appropriate levels, for everything was better
defined than any of the other studies that were carried out, so that while
the big criticism of the Lie study is 9 primary VF's in 106 patients. That
is higher than most other coronary care units would report in its placebo
treatment. Yet when you look over all those studies, it is the best
designed study. It is sort of crazy that someone hasn't done an appropriate study. This is not a long-term study. This is a few day study and
then you have to do life survival analysis and follow-up of the patients,
but probably 2000 patients well studied could answer this question without
any doubt.

Dr. Temple: My comment was only to point out the fact that somebody has
done a pooled analysis doesn't strengthen the data. You are still left
with the Lie study and then all the others.

Dr. Harrison: I didn't show the pooled data for that very reason.

Dr. Campbell: I showed the pooled data for the very reason to knock it
because the pooled data in fact has made the Lie study look more credible
by adding in a lot of other ones and apparently minimizing the effect. I
think it is a dangerous thing to do. The mansucript that I was forced to
produce to come here details in fact 13 studies, mortality rates as opposed
to just the antiarrhythmic effect and in the 13 studies using a variety of
agents including lidocaine obviously, there are 9 which show a modest trend
to improve mortality. There are two studies which show statistically
significant reduction in mortality by prophylactic antiarrhythmic drug
therapy and there, the bad ones again, the Valentine study in Australia
which was hideously skewed in favor of those receiving active therapy and
the study of disopyramide conducted in our country that caused an uproar
and criticism and the results have never been confirmed by anyone else. If
you take these two out, then we are left with very little indeed.

Dr. Temple: One gets the impression that the enthusiasm for lidocaine
has as much to do with its apparent lack of harmfulness as with anybody
being persuaded of its usefulness. What would your view be as the pro-
protagonist of what to do in somebody who doesn't seem to tolerate

lidocaine well. Would you persist with using a second line drug, or would
you abandon the idea at that point because you wouldn't have the very best
tolerated drug available?

Dr. Harrison: I personally would not feel as strong for the second line
drug, but if I were going to use a second line drug at this point in time,
I would probably use procainamide because studies by Koch-Weser and others
showed you could reduce arrhythmias though not VF.

Dr. Sleight: I think, Don you said that the Lie study was terrific. That
sliced bread. It shows it very clearly what I want to show. He used this
very high dose and you didn't actually say that he had something like 17
percent, you know the figures better than I do, but really quite a lot of
severe side effects with that high dose and then you said I reckon it was
more than he needed to use. I think the problem is that there is such a lot
of difficulty in the use of lidocaine properly. If you took a study of the
coronary care units all over the country then you would have a lot of
people poisoned with the stuff, a lot of people totally ineffectively
treated, but a lot of doctors with a placebo effect on their psyche. I
think the doctors have got to learn not to need a placebo effect like that.
I think you have to do that Lie study again.

Dr. Parisi: I would like to ask Dr. Campbell if he ever uses lidocaine
in acute myocardial infarction and if so what are those circumstances?

Dr. Campbell: I do use lidocaine, although I have been sitting here
wondering about tossing this back. I mean the situation in which we use
lidocaine is for the control of a patient who has already shown ventricular
fibrillation and I have been raking out some of the information on how
effective that is. In other words, if you believe this drug is effective,
here is a patient at risk, he has had VF, we know that the electrophysiological mileau that contributed to that is present for sometime afterwards
and the risk of another event of VF is high. But it has been our experience that even with proper doses of lidocaine, that a few of these patients
break through despite what seems optimal therapy. There is a surprising
amount in the literature about this. I am beginning to wonder how useful
lidocaine is even in the prevention of further episodes of ventricular

fibrillation. I am honestly not sure. This drug has an aura that it
works. I take the point that people use it because it seems to be apparently non-toxic. I just don't know if it actually does anything at all.
That is the circumstance in which we use lidocaine for the management of
somebody who has had VF or for a ventricular tachyarrhythmia that is
sustained.

Dr. Copeland: I would like to ask whether we really think the patients
were taken care of in 1983 in the coronary care unit are the same as the
ones we were taking care of when these original studies were done. I think
it is a general rule in a coronary care unit now, patients are on
anywhere from one to three drugs almost from the word go, that includes
nitrates, calcium blockers and beta blockers, and it seems to me that the
incidence of ventricular fibrillation is really not as high now as it used
to be, with or without prophylactic lidocaine. The second thing, is the
incidence of toxicity really the same? I have seen a lot of instances of
heart block that I never saw 10 years ago, when patients are routinely on
calcium blockers and beta blockers especially and are getting lidocaine
prophylaxis in addition to those medications.

Dr. Harrison: All I have to say is that patients in coronary care units
are on many more drugs now and probably there are a larger number of
patients that do not have infarcts that are in the coronary care unit now
than there were 15-20 years ago when the coronary care beds were limited
and a larger percentage of the patients had true infarction in those beds.
All the things the last speaker alluded to I think are true, but I don't
think negate the point of whether or not lidocaine should be used to
prevent primary VF.

Dr.Cohn: Yes and the mortality rate in CCU's is going down and we don't
even know why that is true.

Dr.Campbell: I mean the published evidence on VF rates is that it is
going down precipitously. I mean Lie stands out in having 9% despite his
early admission to CCU. The going rate is now 3 to 4% of primary VF. I
mean the good old days when you could do studies on small numbers of
patients seem to be over.

Dr. Bush: Dr. Goldstein, when you showed the ejection fractions post-recannulation or post-streptokinase, how long after that did you measure ejection fraction?

Dr. Goldstein:: Those ones I showed you were measured immediately afterwards. We have serial data out to 6 months on ejection fraction using radioisotope studies and there was no significant improvement over time.

Dr. Bush: Was it any better at all than the lack of change that you showed in those acute studies?

Dr. Goldstein: There was an unbalancing effect of the radioisotope study. First we went to angiographic studies and then we went to radioisotope studies. I can show that slide, but there was a sort of unbalancing effect so that the groups were not similar, but over time there was no change over the 6 month period.

Dr. Lipicky: How was it that you chose 9 hours to break the data up. Was there some operational way or was that arbitrary?

Dr. Cohn: That was post hoc. We analyzed in all fairness every single interval from the beginning to the end. There was a break point in that all the intervals prior to 9 hours showed a deleterious effect of nitroprusside and every interval we could have chosen after 9 hours showed a beneficial effect. We could have broken it at any one of those points and found the difference betwen the two. We chose 9 hours because the biological data suggested to us that there was a real phenomenon occurring there. It wasn't just a chance clustering. But in all fairness, although time was indeed a consideration when the study was designed, unfortunately we did not randomize with that time interval in mind. So this is post-hoc.

Dr. Lipicky: It seems as though time is a very critical determinant of many outcomes. If one indeed wanted to evaluate whether some kind of early treatment versus some kind of late treatment, or whether there was some kind of pharmacological effect early that was in fact deleterious but beneficial at some later time, indeed, how would one design the trial that could even come close to answering those questions.

158

Dr. Temple: I guess I am not sure that analyzing after the fact for
early and late arrival is necessarily an inadequate way to address that
question. It probably is hard on the spot to stratify that way, given the
emergency nature of most things, I believe it has been tried, but it seems
hard. I am not sure why it is unreasonable to think that treating time
since pain as a covariant is an unreasonable way to approach that question.

Dr. Cohn: The problem in our study Dr. Lipicky is that you had to have
wedge pressure above 12 to get in. Many of the patients who were randomized in the first 8 hours had a wedge pressure above 12. If they had just
by chance arrived at the hospital later, there wedge would have been below
12 and they wouldn't have gotten into the trial at all. It is a totally
different patient population, in addition to them having a different time
interval.

Dr. Temple: I think you should do it prospectively.

Dr. Cohn: Yes, you should do it prospectively.

Dr. Lipicky: I don't know whether this is right or not, but the thing
that disturbed me a little bit in terms of thinking of retrospective
analysis of time is that although you rather flat-footedly said that at
every interval of time, the treated group was worse than the placebo, in
all probability you couldn't really draw that conclusion because the
populations that you had, the numbers that you had at these other time
slices were too small.

Dr. Cohn: They were small, but we are talking about 800 patient study and
after you start subdividing them, they get small numbers but we are not
talking about 5 and 6 patients. There were 20-40 patients in these groups.

Dr. Ruberio: Assuming that the mortality in acute phase of MI is 15%
and assuming that I have a drug that can reduce the mortality by 20%. What
does it mean to reduce the mortality from 15% to 12%? Nothing might do
that, and if I have to design a trial that has a statistical power of 90%
and I am looking for a p value less than .05, I need approximately 3800
patients randomized to either control or treated groups, and I don't think

that anybody will be at this moment of the game, willing to do that number of patients. So my question to Dr. Temple is, if someone wants to have a claim in reduction of infarct size, what is the position of the FDA. Are you looking for difference in mortality or would you be evaluating interactive parameters in order to provide the claim.

Dr. Temple: That is a good question. I don't completely have the answer. I think one has to be struck by the observation that every time you use an end point that wasn't really what you wanted to know, you run the risk of making a mistake. As you probably know, intracoronary streptokinase is an approved agent. It was approved on the basis on the clear showing that it dissolved clots. Now there is clearly a reasonable degree of question as to whether it is beneficial and perhaps even whether it might be harmful. Anytime that you take the end point that really wasn't what you really wanted, you run that risk. Other examples could be cholesterol lowering agents and a variety of other things. I guess my feeling is that even though a study like that involves a large number of people, it doesn't necessarily require very prolonged intense observation. It requires a brief period of intense observation and then a relatively easy kind of follow up which consists of finding out whether they are alive or dead. That is comparatively easy and in fact trials of that kind are going on now, so they are not impossible. That is part 1 of the answer. The second part would be how much concensus one could obtain on how you should measure reduction infarct size. If it became very persuasive I guess that some kind of measurement really corresponded to something meaningful, it would be easier to conclude that an apparent reduction in infarct size was a reasonable measure, but you would still have the nagging question of whether , for example someone this morning said you are producing a more at risk area of myocardium. I mean if there is such a thing as a swiss-cheese infarct and if those cells are permanently ready to go off, you haven't done a person good by salvaging this little bit of myocardium. My own bias in this, subject to concensus building and other arguments is that where it can be done, and it can be done, you can think of a study to do this, probably the thing that you really want to know which is preferably mortality but certainly if not that, some reasonable measure of myocardial performance. That might be a reasonable end point.

Dr. Ruberio: I would like to ask Dr. Rentrop. Your group with nitroglycerine was the only one that showed an improvement in ejection fraction, is
that correct?

Dr. Rentrop: Only the patients that received streptokinase showed improvement.

Dr. Ruberio: What do you think is the potential for the tissue plasminogen activator if you see any?

Dr. Rentrop: Conceptually it is a very interesting and tantalizing drug
since it should avoid some of the problems that we have with intravenous
streptokinase and possibly be more efficacious. There are problems to it
from a practical point of view. So far the question of a
production at a reasonable price and in large enough quantities seems to be
unsolved and I don't know of anybody who confidentially can predict when it
would be solved. Secondly, the availablility also may be a problem.
Apparently the substance disappears very quickly from the circulation and
the question needs to be answered whether it will be bound to the clot in
sufficient quantity in that short interval. It probably gets back to the
price question. Yes it is an interesting drug, but as to its practical
availability, we don't know the answers yet.

Dr. Temple: Dr. Cohn, you showed the dramatic influence of what I took
to be the initial measurement of filling pressure on mortality. You didn't
break that slide down into before 9 hours and after 9 hours, but in your
summary wrap up explanation, you said that there is a big difference in
prognosis depending upon whether the wedge pressure is up early or up late.
What do the mortality values look like in the placebo group if you break it
down that way.

Dr. Cohn: The mortality placebo-nitroprusside by hours data show that
break and the trends are about the same actually for the placebo group.

Dr. Temple: Doesn't that call your explanation into some question?

Dr. Cohn: Because?

Dr. Temple: The hypothesis is that an elevated wedge pressure early has no particular prognostic significance because it is just going to fix itself, which I thought was the explanation. If none-the-less in the placebo group, an elevated wedge pressure early corresponds to a very high mortality, then it looks like it has the same significance as it has with a late elevated wedge pressure.

Dr. Cohn: You are right to a certain extent about that but it has to do with the magnitude of the increase. That is the group that falls usually begins with modest elevations. You will notice the break in that was 18 and below and then 18 to 22 and above 22. The real high mortality is in the group that is above 18 and above 22 and those don't tend to fall so much. There is some discrepancy, which is why I don't discourage the use of vasodilators in the first few hours in somebody whose wedge pressure is above 22. You will notice that the mortality was not increased in that group by nitroprusside either. The data really have to be analyzed in a lot more detail and you are quite right that that one slide lumps a lot of things together, taking all comers, the wedge pressure is a very important determinant.

Dr. Goldstein: Didn't the drug study show that it didn't make any difference what the wedge pressure was?

Dr. Cohn: They didn't have wedge pressures.

Dr. Goldstein: They just took all comers.

Dr. Cohn: They took all comers and they titrated nitroprusside to lowering of the blood pressure to 110 or as close to 100 as they could get it, and they used a much higher dose of nitroprusside. We of course titrated nitroprusside to lower the wedge pressure. Our goal was to lower the wedge, not to lower the blood pressure. They got a beneficial effect which kind of surprised everybody, because that is not the way most people use nitroprusside in acute MI. We then subsequently re-analyzed our data and looking at those patients whose pressures were dropped below 110 to try to amass to a certain extent the Netherlands data and the mortality is always higher in those whose pressure falls to below 110 during either placebo or

nitroprusside than in those whose pressure doesn't fall so much so I see no
evidence that the further lowering of blood pressure had a favorable
effect.

Karin Heller: I have a question for Dr. Rentrop. In your preliminary data
from the Mount Sinai, New York University Study you showed that the streptokinase had a positive effect on the echocardiogram, but it looked from your
data as if a combination of streptokinase and nitroglycerine had a negative
effect. I was wondering how you would explain those results?

Dr. Rentrop: I can't. The numbers are fairly small and we are talking
about p value of .05 so it is not that strong. We will have to see if that
holds up in the future. I could speculate that these patients got intravenous nitroglycerine following the intracoronary infusion of nitroglycerine
and that maybe we did bad things to pressure and that these type lesions
that persist at recannulization did not allow sufficient perfusion in the
presence of nitroglycerine afterwards, but that is pure conjecture and I
don't know the answer.

Dr. Tuzel: My question is similar to what Dr. Temple asked, but this is
in relation to age. You mentioned that age is also one of the predictors
of mortality. For those patients who were given nitroprusside less than 9
hours, was there an age differential? Was that taken into account? When
you reach your conclusion that it might be detrimental, was there a difference in age?

Dr. Cohn: We stratified for age in our trial and there was no difference
based upon age and the response to nitroprusside. I have no idea, I wish
somebody could tell me why the older you are, the more likely you are to
die from an acute myocardial infarction. We all know that that is true.
Even when you correct for every other factor such as the wedge pressure,
and the previous infarct, and previous history of heart failure and everything that you sort of associate with age, you find that age hangs out as
an independent determinant of survival. Interestingly enough, when you
look at congestive heart failure, there is absolutely no influence of age
on mortality and congestive heart failure.

Dr. Goldstein: It depends upon the weight of the event. If you look at congestive heart failure it obviously overwhelms everything else around. I think that you can statistically "control" for those events, but they are probably manifestations of other things that you can't control. I think when you take an older age group population as compared to a younger one, you can control for all sorts of things, but those are only tips of many icebergs in a pathological field that are coming up at you.

Dr. Dern: In regard to the question of dealing from time of onset of problems and the issue of going back over the data and looking at it and breaking up the data you know at 9 hours, I think one suggestion that I have is that if one had previous information, let's say that time from onset of ischemia was important, that one could instead of inspecting the data and then picking 9 hours, lets say take some type of unbiased, let's take the median time from onset of chest pain. That is not biased by the inspection, one could look at the median. One could look at the group up above and below the median. That is not based on any inspection of the data but it is based on an idea that there are obviously two groups there and one has not determined that by inspection, and then within each of those groups perform an analysis adjusting for a few other variables, let's say age plus ejection fraction. This might give you such strongly significant p values that in fact you are finding on time from infarct or from time of onset of ischemia might be useful. In other words, even though it was retrospective in one sense, the p value might be so strong that you would accept that you had a demonstration of effect of time. In think this is another thing one can do, but it is based on some notion, probably in the beginning of the appropriate time to do this and in the absence of that time and if you don't want to get in trouble from inspection of the data, then we'll take it at the median.

Dr. Cohn: I appreciate your suggestions but I am not sure how to analyze it at this point. The problem of course with that is that if there really is a biological event occurring and the time is very critical, you may so hide the data by choosing inappropriate time, that you won't find the differences that you set out to look for.

Dr. Goldstein: Apropo to Dr. Lipicky's question, I think that there are a

number of events going on in the acute infarction period and I think it is
important to separate those out. I think there is some type of acute event
going on. Whether that is an infarct, low flow state thrombis, or an
akinetic segment that goes on to infarction. There is a period of time
when that occurs. I think it occurs very early, probably within the first
few minutes. Thombosis clearly is a major event at that time. There is
probably some sort of quiescent period, or at least a fall off in the
event, and then one begins seeing new events occurring, probably beginning
with that event, but probably building up to sometime around 6 to 12 hours
after infarction. I think then you are looking at a whole new constella-
tion of events and I think as was suggested this morning, that there are
probable microinfarcts, or multiple small infarcts going on in the post-
infarct period. I don't think we can deal with the acute event in the
sense of changing infarct size and I think that is our observation in the
streptokinase studies where unless you really are there within minutes, the
clinical events have become so dominant that there is nothing you can
effect. But you can effect the later events. I think those are very
important events. They are not to be underestimated. In our observations
that streptokinase seemed to make the collateral bed look better, for
instance the aspirin trial in unstable angina seemed to decrease the events
of reinfarction in people with unstable angina, I think are all impressive
to suggest that there are lots of events going on after the major presenting event, whatever that is, and I think that is really where we ought to
develop our approaches of interventions. Whether this is a beta blocker or
whether it is something like a specific agent which will prevent lyse
thrombus in the tissue, in the coronary arteries.

Dr. Rentrop: I think I disagree with your fatalistic approach to the
first minutes and hours of infarction, but before spelling that out, I
would like to ask you, would you care to comment on Anderson's findings
which you failed to mention in your discussion.

Dr. Goldstein: I think that the Anderson data obviously didn't support my
premise, so that I was why I didn't use it. I used your slide, that was
bad enough. I wouldn't want to be critical of other investigators, but I
think the Anderson study was clouded by a number of issues, one of which is
that patients were not randomized after angiography. Secondly they

included a number of people who did not have total occlusions, and that
makes it difficult to understand what streptokinase was doing in people who
did not have total occlusion. They talked about restitution reperfusion of
vessels which were already opened prior to the administration of
streptokinase, so I have a little difficulty in that. I had some
difficulty with the methodology of looking at infarct size in that study.
I think all of the techniques that they used are open for a lot of
question, including our own.

Dr. Rentrop: Yes, I personally think it is not correct, but I would not
exclude patients with septal lesions like you did. I actually think it
probably is not even correct to randomize only after angiography because at
that point a lot of things have happened already which may very well
influence outcome and your entering the patients into the study at this
point may be quite biased and exclude important segments of the population.
Aside from that the main issue I think when we compare your trial and
Anderson's trial as pointed by Swan and the accompanying editorial, the
difference in duration of symptoms between the two trials.

Dr. Goldstein: Clearly, theirs were one hour earlier and I would not
minimize one hour earlier, but I think one hour between hour 3 and hour 2
would be very important or one hour as you showed very nicely on your slide
that one hour change is really critical. One hour at times 4 and 5 I think
is probably not as critical. Others have used a mean arrival time of 4
hours as compared to our 5.4 which is actually shorter than the Anderson
study and they found the same thing we did. I don't think that time frame
is important. I would grant you that if they were getting into hour 2 or 3
that would be critical.

Dr. Rentrop: Some have had a very poor reperfusion rate and a very high
re-occlusion rate. I think that is a study which shows poor technique,
that is all it shows, and that poor technique doesn't work. Quite frankly,
I think that none of these studies that are in are really strong enough to
say either it works or it doesn't work at this point and I guess everyone
remains entitled to his bias and my bias still is that very early reperfusion at least in large infarcts does work, and if it does work, then you
said "So what, because we don't get the patients early enough". But here

is where I would not accept such a fatalistic approach. If it should be found to work, logistics can be organized, patients can be educated, and that has been shown in various communities in Seattle and in Berlin where education in the public resulted in drastic shortening of time between onset of symptom and hospital admission. If it is worth it, I think it should be attempted and we should not be so fatalistic.

Dr. Goldstein: I agree with Dr. Rentrop that certainly reperfusion is to be aspired to and I think it is possible. I think we responded to a wave of enthusiasm that you can reperfuse almost the next day and I think that probably is nonsense. But on the other hand, it would be wonderful to do it in the first couple hours. I am not as enthusiastic as you are about educating people. We studied the arrival time of people to the coronary care unit in Rochester, N.Y. in 1965 and average time was 6 hours. Almost 20 years later, it is still 6 hours in almost every country it has been studied in around the world. Now granted emergency care units get to bedsides faster for cardiac arrest, but the arrival time of the patient to the coronary care unit is still in the 4 to 6 hour range. It is still outside the range that we can make any meaningful intervention.

Dr. Cohn: Intrinsic to a lot of the study with thrombolysis of course is the concept of whether the clot is really the cause of acute myocardial infarctions. I guess it doesn't exclude the fact that the clot may come later and still have an effect on the course, but I wonder what the view is of the panel. How many on the panel harbor any questions in their minds, as to whether most myocardial and transmural MI's are caused by clots. Anybody question that.

Dr. Rentrop: I am quite sure it is a secondary.

Dr. Campbell: I question it. There is no doubt that the evidence from patients who die of sudden death, the incidence of clot is low, although many of these may in fact be the patients who are worthy to survive that incident, wouldn't go on to show evidence of infarction. Now that I have something to say, I was just musing whether clinical ventricular fibrilla-tion seen in the coronary care unit may not be something very good and obviously represent reperfusion. We shouldn't view ventricular fibrillation as necessarily a bad thing.

Dr. Goldstein: Dr. Rentrop, you think the clot is the primary event, yes or no.

Dr. Rentrop: As a matter of fact, I would like to learn how I am supposed not to think that.

Dr. Goldstein: How many people in the audience harbor any questions as to whether the clot is primary event. How many people are concerned that the clot may not be primary event, just to get some idea. (Many hands are raised). O.K. everybody is not convinced about this and I think that very vital to our ongoing understanding of the syndrome and where we should be putting most of our emphasis. It may be quite right that the clot starts that process, but we still have to convince some skeptics.

16

EARLY INTRAVENOUS ATENOLOL IN SUSPECTED ACUTE MYOCARDIAL
INFARCTION: FINAL REPORT OF A RANDOMISED CLINICAL TRIAL

S. YUSUF, D. RAMSDALE, P. SLEIGHT, P. ROSSI, R. PETO,
M. PEARSON, H. STERRY, L. FURSE, R. MOTWANI, S. PARISH,
R. GRAY, D. BENNETT, C. BRAY

INTRODUCTION

The amount of myocardial damage following infarction is
an important predictor of morbidity and mortality.[1,2]   In
experimental infarction beta-adrenergic blocking agents
have been shown to reduce infarct size when given to animals
prior to or soon after coronary artery ligation.[3]   However,
several trials of _oral_ beta-blockers in acute myocardial
infarction (MI) have failed to show any beneficial effect on
infarct size,[4] arrhythmias[5] or mortality,[6-8] perhaps partly
because some of these oral trials included patients presenting
late after pain, and partly because there may be a substantial
delay between the administration of oral treatment and the
achievement of adequate beta-blockade.[9]   An _early intravenous_
dose is needed for rapid adequate beta-blockade.[10]

We have previously reported the preliminary results from
the first 214 patients admitted to our randomised, controlled
study of the effects of early intravenous beta-blockade on
infarct size.[11]   There was then a marginally significant
reduction in ECG and enzyme indices of infarct size. The
complete study includes 477 patients with suspected acute MI,
randomised at an average of 5 hours of the onset of symptoms to
receive either standard management, or immediate intravenous
atenolol followed by 10 days of oral treatment. Our main aim
was to discover the effects of this schedule on:

> (i)   the ECG and enzyme estimates of eventual
>   infarct size among patients who already,
>   prior to randomisation, had ECG evidence
>   suggestive of recent infarction (the

'definite MI'[11] group of 307 patients), and

(ii) the probability of certain indices of infarction
      eventually developing among the patients whose
      pre-randomisation ECGs did not provide such
      evidence (the 'threatened MI'[11] group of
      170 patients).

Our secondary aim was to compare the clinical course, ancillary
drug therapy, morbidity and mortality of treated and control
patients.

PATIENTS AND METHODS

These are as described in our previous report,[11] except
that the full period of intake now runs from August 1978 to
May 1981. Patients with a clinical history strongly suggestive
of myocardial infarction within the previous 12 hours were
considered eligible whether or not ECG abnormalities had already
become evident. Formal criteria for exclusion included heart rate
less than 40 beats/min; systolic BP less than 90 mm Hg; second
degree or greater heart block; heart failure requiring digoxin or
more than 80 mg of frusemide; or a history of asthma. Patients
already on a beta-blocker and patients thought to require
immediate beta-blockade (e.g. for hypertension) were ineligible,
as were any patients in whom it was suspected on informal
clinical criteria that beta-blockade was contraindicated. This
meant that no randomised patients had an initial systolic BP below
100 mm Hg, and only 2% had an initial heart rate below 50.
During most of the trial no formal list of the causes of
exclusion was maintained, but in a sample period they were due
in approximately similar proportions to current beta-blockade,
late (>12 hours) presentation, and contraindications. About a
quarter of all acute MI admissions to the coronary care units
remained eligible, and of these probably just over half were
randomised.

Procedure for randomisation

Numbered, sealed envelopes were used for randomisation.
Name, heart rate, blood pressure and time from onset of pain were
recorded on the envelope before it was opened to prevent

foreknowledge of the randomised group and unauthorised withdrawal
Once an envelope was opened the patient was irrevocably in the
trial, even where admission criteria were not fully met (i.e.
3 patients admitted more than 12 hours after onset of pain).

Three minor problems arose as a result of the involvement
of resident staff unfamiliar with randomised trials that could
have been avoided by telephoned randomisation. Envelopes were
occasionally used out of order, but this did not cause bias.
An envelope opened for one patient was reused for two later
patients. Only the first patient is regarded as having been
entered into the trial (although inclusion of the two excluded
patients would scarcely change our findings). Eleven envelopes
(4 atenolol, 7 control, with widely scattered envelope numbers)
were not accounted for. Search of the CCU logs between the
opening dates of previous and subsequent numbered envelopes did
not suggest that patients had been entered and then removed from
the trial. None of the collaborating physicians know of
occasions on which second envelopes were improperly opened in the
hope of changing an unwanted allocation for an unusual patient
and patients on the subsequent envelopes were not unusual.
Moreover, excluding them from all analyses did not materially
alter our findings.

Treatment

Patients randomised to therapy immediately received
5 mg atenolol intravenously (slowly over 5 minutes). If no undue
hypotension or bradycardia was apparent, oral doses of 50 mg
were given immediately and 12 hrs later, with 100 mg once daily
thereafter for 10 days or until the patient developed
contraindications, died or was discharged. Control patients did
not receive placebos, and were allowed beta-blockade if this was
clearly indicated. Routine ancillary management of the patients
was not intended to be much altered by the study protocol (but
see results section below), and was not under the direct control
of the investigators. Post mortems were not routinely performed,
so in most cases pathological causes of death are not available.

Enzyme and ECG measurements

At entry 8 ml of blood was drawn for enzyme estimations.

Subsequent samples were drawn 4-hourly for the next 48 hrs
and 6-hourly for the next 24 hrs, except in the middle of the
third night. The plasma was separated, stored at $-20^{\circ}C$, and
analysed for total CKMB (the MB isomer of creatinine kinase)
without knowledge of treatment and clinical details. Cumulative
CKMB was calculated for each patient by a modification[12] of the
method of Sobel et al.[1]

Standard 12 lead ECGs were recorded before randomisation,
on the 3rd day, and at discharge, and were measured as described
elsewhere.[13] Patients were subdivided into two groups based on
a 'blind' reading of the initial ECG:

Group 1 (the 'definite MI' group) - Evidence on the
pre-randomisation ECG suggestive of recent infarction, i.e. ST
segment elevation of at least 1 mm in the limb leads or 2 mm in
the praecordial leads[11,14] (with or without Q waves).

Group 2 (the 'threatened MI' group) - All others. Group 2
patients were further subdivided into Group 2a, i.e. those whose
pre-randomisation ECG was suggestive of some abnormality
(e.g. T wave inversion, ST depression or bundle branch
block (BBB) on the initial ECG), and Group 2b, i.e. those with
no abnormality apparent on their pre-randomisation ECG.

Definition of 'eventual' infarction and reinfarction

Patients were classified as having developed an infarct
if, during the 10 days after randomisation, they showed more
than a 20% reduction in their 'R-wave score' (see below) or
produced a cumulative enzyme output of at least twice the
upper limit of the normal range for CKMB (i.e. cumulative
values of at least 10 IU). These criteria differ from those
used to separate groups 1 and 2 at entry.

If after the first 3 days patients developed any two of the
following they were considered to have reinfarcted:
characteristic chest pain, further R-wave loss, renewed enzyme
elevation.

R-wave score

ECG evolution during the days after randomisation was
interpreted using an index that we called the 'R-wave score'.[11]
This compares the worst of the later ECGs with the

pre-randomisation ECG, and expresses the size of the R-waves in certain leads[11] as a percentage of their size in the pre-randomisation ECG. This score was about 100% for patients who suffered no infarction and 0% for patients whose R-waves disappeared in all such leads. Since this score could not be assessed reliably for patients with persistent bundle branch block (BBB) or major axis deviations, or for patients dying before a final ECG was recorded, our scoring system was arbitrarily extended as follows:

1. Death within 10 days - score defined as 0%.
2. Persistent right or left BBB or major axis deviation initially, with no further worsening of the ECG - score defined as 100%.
3. Persistent right or left BBB or major axis deviation developing after entry - score arbitrarily defined either as 25%, or as 10% if both developed.

Statistical methods

Long-term (1-4 years, thus far) follow-up for mortality was obtained by 'flagging' patients through the National Health Service Central Registry, courtesy of the Office of Population Censuses and Surveys.

It was initially planned to randomise 200 patients, but calculations based on the degree of variation of the cumulative CKMB (but not on the apparent treatment effect) among the first 100 patients suggested that at least 400 patients would be needed to detect even a 33% reduction in infarct size reasonably reliably. Recruitment was therefore extended to May 1981, by which time 477 patients had been randomised and another study was beginning.

Data have been expressed as mean $\pm$ standard error of mean, with standard confidence intervals for certain effects. Continuous variables were analysed using standard 't'-tests* and

---

*To check on the accuracy of estimating P-values by t-tests for the effects of treatment on enzyme release, all such P-values were also re-calculated (a) after logarithmic transformation (taking all values below 10 IU as equivalent to 10 IU), (b) by permutational arguments, and (c) both, but in no case was the P-value materially altered.

discrete variables using standard chi-square tests; all P values
are two-tailed (2P).

RESULTS

  Some clinical details of the initial condition of the
patients are given in Table 1. The two groups were comparable
for all entry variables except maleness, diabetes, and previous
history of MI, all of which were non-significantly commoner
in the treated group. The mean time from the onset of symptoms
to randomisation was relatively short (5 hrs) in both groups and
88% of the patients were entered within 8 hrs.

Table 1. Condition at entry

	Nos. of patients/mean values	
	ATENOLOL	CONTROLS
Total randomised	244	233
Women	30	43 (NS)
Age (years)	56	56
Systolic BP (mm Hg)	143	145
Diastolic BP (mm Hg)	89	91
Heart rate (bpm)	77	77
No. with BBB/major axis deviation	11	9
PR interval at entry (sec)	0.16	0.16
Heart failure at entry	15	16
Previous history of:		
Angina	25	29
Hypertension	29	28
Myocardial infarction	44	34 (NS)
Diabetes	14	9 (NS)
Site of myocardial infarction:		
Anterior	100	91
Inferior	86	86
Both	12	5
Indefinite	46	51
Time from pain to randomisation:		
Mean (hrs)	5.0	5.0
≤ 2 hours	13	24
$>2 \leq 4$ "	99	81
$>4 \leq 6$ "	67	62
$>6 \leq 8$ "	37	34
$>8 \leq 13$ "	27	31
Unknown	1	1

NS = not significant (2P> 0.05)

Results among patients presenting with only threatened infarction (Group 2)

One hundred and seventy patients had only 'threatened' infarction at entry (Table 2). Of these, 49% of the atenolol group and 66% of the controls subsequently developed infarction.

Table 2. Eventual infarction during 10-day treatment period among patients with only threatened infarction at entry

Group no. & characteristic	ATENOLOL eventual infarct / threatened infarct		CONTROLS eventual infarct / threatened infarct	
2a Suspicious ECG initially	31/51	(61%)	45/60	(75%)
2b Normal ECG initially	6/25	(24%)	17/34	(50%)
2 Total	37/76	(49%)	62/94	(66%)

Test for effect, combining information from 2a and 2b: $X_1^2 = 6.2$, P<0.02

This suggests prevention of progression to infarction in about one-sixth of Group 2 patients, but because the effect is only moderately significant ($X^2 = 6.2$, 2P<0.02) the confidence limits for its true magnitude are wide, so the true proportion protected could be as much as two-sixths or it could be negligible (although the clear reduction in infarct size reported below in Group 1 suggests some real effect in Group 2). The mean cumulative CKMB release in Group 2 was slightly but not significantly lower in the treated patients (25 $\pm$ 6 IU) than in the controls (32 $\pm$ 5 IU), and the mean R-wave score was significantly (t = 2.32; 2P<0.02) better in treated patients (87 $\pm$ 3%) than in controls (78 $\pm$ 3%) (Figs. 1 & 2). When the patients with threatened infarction were subdivided by initial heart rate, ECG status, blood pressure, time from randomisation or site of infarction (anterior/other), there was no clear

evidence that the protection against eventual infarction was
different in different subgroups.

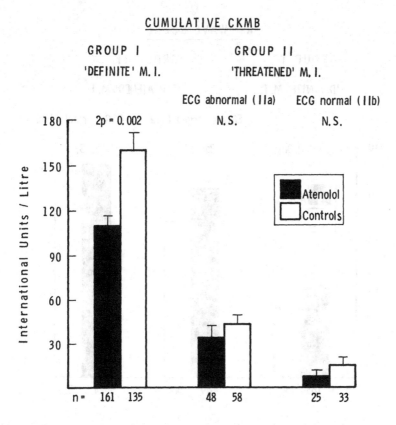

FIGURE 1.   Cumulative CKMB release in patients with initial
'definite' ECG changes (Group 1), initial 'suspicious' ECG changes
(Group 2a) and an initial normal ECG (Group 2b).   Standard errors
are indicated.

Results among patients presenting with 'definite' infarction
(Group 1)

Three hundred and seven patients were classified as having
'definite' infarction at entry, 168 of whom received atenolol.
Except for one patient in the atenolol group, all had definite
MI confirmed by subsequent ECG or enzyme changes.

Enzyme data were available in 296 of the 307 patients (96%),
of whom 161 were randomised to receive atenolol.   The mean
cumulative enzyme release was 109.9 IU/1 $\pm$ 8.1 in the atenolol

group compared to 160.3 IU/l ± 13.8 in the control group
(t = 3.27; 2P = 0.001) (Fig. 1). This ratio of 0.69 suggests a
decrease of about one-third in enzyme release, but with a standard

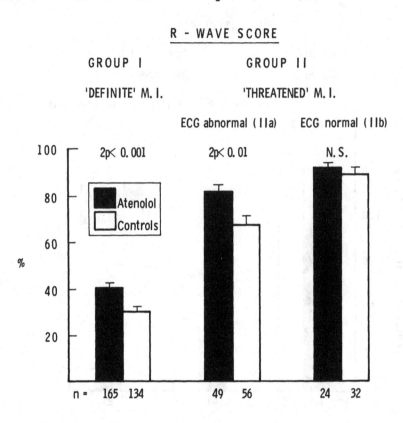

FIGURE 2. R-wave score in patients with initial 'definite' ECG
changes (Group 1), initial 'suspicious' ECG changes (Group 2a)
and an initial normal ECG (Group 2b). Standard errors are
indicated.

95% confidence interval for the fractional decrease ranging from
one-sixth to one-half. Patients were subdivided by initial heart
rate, blood pressure, time from randomisation, site of infarction
and age, as in Group 2. Again, there was no clear evidence that
the degree of protection was materially different in different
such subgroups, for in each the patients treated with atenolol had
less enzyme release than their respective control patients
(Fig. 3).

<u>Complete R-wave data</u> were available for 299 of the
307 Group 1 patients (97%). The mean R-wave score was 41.1% ± 2.0
in the atenolol group and 30.7% ± 2.1 in the controls (t = 3.56;

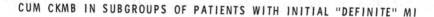

CUM CKMB IN SUBGROUPS OF PATIENTS WITH INITIAL "DEFINITE" MI

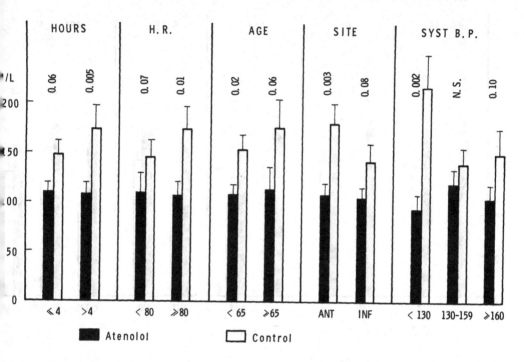

FIGURE 3. Cumulative CKMB release in Group 1 patients
divided into various subgroups based on time from onset of pain
to entry, initial heart rate, age, site of infarction
(anterior/other - chiefly inferior) and systolic blood pressure.
Standard errors are indicated.

2P<0.001) (Fig. 2), suggesting better myocardial preservation in
the treated than in the control group. When these Group 1
patients were subdivided in various ways (as above), the mean
R-wave scores were always higher in the treated patients than in
their corresponding controls (Fig. 4).
<u>Clinical course, morbidity and mortality (Groups 1 and 2)</u>
Mortality data are available for all patients, but all data
on clinical course and morbidity are missing in one atenolol and

two control patients.

R-WAVE SCORE IN SUBGROUPS OF PATIENTS WITH INITIAL "DEFINITE" MI

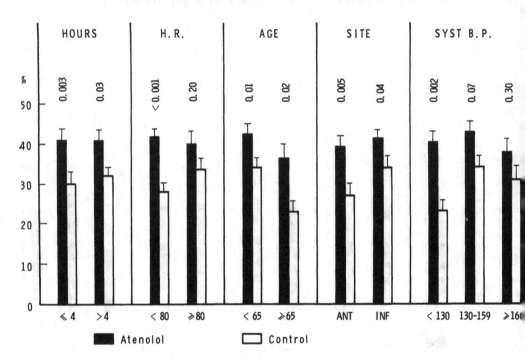

FIGURE 4.   R-wave score in Group 1 patients divided into various subgroups based on time from onset of pain to entry, initial heart rate, age, site of infarction (anterior/other - chiefly inferior) and systolic blood pressure.   Standard errors are indicated.

Heart failure and conduction delay (Tables 3 and 4).   Table 3 describes the incidence, severity and treatment of heart failure in the two groups.   Radiological evidence (as assessed by routine radiological reports) of heart failure was seen in 24% of control and 19% of treated patients.   The more severe changes of pulmonary and interstitial oedema were twice as common in the control group (15% vs 7%).   These benefits were reflected in a significantly lower dose requirement of loop-diuretics and digoxin in the treated patients.   Although there was no increase

Table 3. Heart failure, diuretics and digoxin during 10-day treatment period

	Nos. of patients	
	ATENOLOL	CONTROLS
Total randomised	244	233
Radiological evidence of heart failure:		
At entry	15	16
After entry:		
(a) Mild (pulmonary congestion/ upper lobe diversion)	28	22
(b) Moderate/severe (pulmonary oedema/interstitial oedema)	18	34*
(c) Total	46	56
Treatment for heart failure in hospital:		
Loop diuretic	93	89
Mean dose (equivalent[+] dose of frusemide in mg) & standard error of mean	149±19	205±32*
Other diuretics	40	55*
Digoxin	16	31*
Drugs at discharge:		
Diuretic at discharge	66	57 (NS)
Digoxin at discharge	11	20 (NS)

[+]A few patients received bumetanide, and for this calculation 1 mg of bumetanide = 40 mg of frusemide.

*$0.01 < 2P < 0.05$;

 NS = not statistically significant ($2P > 0.05$)

in the number of patients with A-V nodal conduction delay, the PR interval showed a small but significant prolongation in treated patients. The reduction in bundle branch block and major axis deviation in the treated group may have been related to decreased myocardial damage (Table 4).

Table 4. Selected findings during 10-day treatment period

	Nos. of patients/mean values $\pm$ SE	
	ATENOLOL (244)	CONTROLS (233)
(a) ARRHYTHMIAS		
Atrial fibrillation	12 (5%)**	29 (12%)
Atrial flutter	4	7
Supraventricular tachycardia	13	23
Any supraventricular arrhythmia (i.e. any of above)	28 (11%)*	45 (19%)
Accelerated idioventricular rhythm	41	40
Ventricular tachycardia	39 (NS)	52
(b) BUNDLE BRANCH BLOCK (BBB) AND HEART BLOCK		
BBB/major axis deviation at entry	11	9
BBB/major axis deviation after randomisation	16 (7%)*	28 (12%)
PR interval $\geq$0.20 sec at entry	45	44
Heart block after randomisation:		
I$^{\circ}$	34	32
II$^{\circ}$	2	8
III$^{\circ}$	11	10
Sinus arrest	5 (NS)	1
Mean PR interval (sec) at entry	0.163 $\pm$ 0.002	0.162 $\pm$ 0.002
Mean PR interval (sec) after entry	0.165 $\pm$ 0.002^{+}	0.159 $\pm$ 0.002
Temporary pacemaker	11	12
(c) OTHER FINDINGS		
Bradycardia	43 (18%)*	24 (10%)
Hypotension	60 (25%)**	34 (15%)
Cardiogenic shock	1 (NS)	4
Atropine	23	19
Inotropic agents	4	6

**2P<0.01, *2P<0.05, NS = not statistically significant (2P>0.05)

$^{+}$t = 2.04*. If the changes in PR interval are assessed by a paired t-test, the differences cease to be statistically significant. Initial PR interval is unavailable in 16 atenolol and 14 control patients due to a variety of reasons, e.g. atrial fibrillation, etc.

Cardiac arrhythmias (Table 4). There was a marginally significant reduction in the incidence of supraventricular arrhythmias (2P<0.03) in treated patients, the effect being most marked for atrial fibrillation (2P<0.01). Although this suggests a direct antiarrhythmic effect, it may be merely secondary to a decrease in myocardial damage. There was no increase in the incidence of accelerated idioventricular rhythm, despite the slower heart rate that beta-blockade produces. There was a non-significant tendency for ventricular tachycardia to be observed less frequently, the direction of which is consistent with our experience with continuous tape-recording in the first 24 hrs.[15]

Cardiac arrest and mortality (Table 5). Fewer treated patients suffered cardiac arrest (Table 5). Many of these arrests occurred only after the patients had been transferred from the CCU to the ordinary wards, and so were not on ECG monitors. Thus it is uncertain whether these episodes were due to ventricular fibrillation or asystole. Three control patients developed recurrent cardiac arrest and died in hospital, and 3 other control patients arrested and died unexpectedly without prior heart failure or recurrent chest pain, making a total of 6 control and no treated patients who arrested and died in the first 10 days. In addition, 7 treated and 10 control patients died in other circumstances during the first 10 days, so total in-hospital mortality was only marginally significantly reduced (7 vs 16). Pooling non-fatal cardiac arrest and/or death within 10 days, the difference becomes more significant (11 atenolol vs 25 controls; 2P = 0.01). This suggests that the odds of developing a major cardiac event are approximately halved, but of course the corresponding confidence limits are extremely wide, so the true magnitude of any such reduction cannot be predicted reliably.

Table 5. Reinfarction, cardiac arrest and mortality during 10-day treatment period, and later mortality

	Nos. of patients	
	ATENOLOL	CONTROLS
Total randomised	244	233
REINFARCTION IN HOSPITAL	O	6
CARDIAC ARREST AND/OR DEATH:		
1. Non-fatal cardiac arrest*: patient alive at day 10	4	9
2. Non-fatal cardiac arrest: patient dead at day 10	O	3
3. Fatal cardiac arrest by day 10 without prior heart failure or recurrent chest pain	O	3
ALL CARDIAC ARRESTS[+] (sum of 1-3)	4	15^1
4. Other deaths by day 10	7	10
ALL DEATHS BY DAY 10 (sum of 2-4)	7	16^2
DEATH AND/OR ARREST BY DAY 10 (sum of 1-4)	11	25^3
5. Death recorded after day 10 in relation to number of survivors at day 10	29/237 (12.2%)	27/217 (12.4%)
TOTAL DEATHS RECORDED	36	43

*1 and 2 of these respectively were fast VTs requiring defibrillation.

[+]After 10 days 1 further arrest was recorded, bringing the total number of cardiac arrests to 4 and 16.

$1\chi^2 = 8.2$, $2P<0.008$

$2\chi^2 = 4.1$, $2P<0.05$

$3\chi^2 = 6.6$, $2P<0.01$

After the end of the drug treatment at day 10, we have 1-4 years of follow-up, during which time we have learned of 27/217 (12.4%) control and 29/237 (12.2%) treated deaths.

Adverse effects (Table 4). As expected, bradycardia and hypotension were more common in the treated group than in the control group, but these should generally be viewed as main effects of treatment, rather than adverse effects. The number of patients receiving atropine was similar in the two groups, suggesting that most instances of bradycardia associated with atenolol were adequately treated by stopping atenolol. Similarly, there was no difference in the use of inotropic agents or the incidence of cardiogenic shock (but see Discussion).

Ancillary drug treatment in hospital. Fewer atenolol-treated patients required antihypertensive agents (58 vs 76; 2P<0.03), other antiarrhythmic drugs (14 vs 41; 2P<0.001) or calcium-channel blocking agents (9 vs 22; 2P<0.02). The use of oral anticoagulants, antiplatelet agents and bronchodilators was similar in the two groups.

Protocol deviations

Three patients randomised to the atenolol group did not receive intravenous or oral beta-blocker, and 2 control patients did receive intravenous beta-blocker. All analyses include these 5 'deviants' in their original allocated group (i.e. are 'intention to treat' analyses). During the 10-day trial period, oral beta-blockade was instituted among 44 controls and discontinued in 75 atenolol-allocated patients. These changes chiefly affected beta-blockade after infarction was largely completed, and although they may have diluted any treatment effects on reinfarction they should not necessarily be thought of as protocol deviations - indeed, from the outset it was envisaged that, on intentionally imprecise clinical grounds, oral beta-blockade should be used whenever it was advisable (e.g. for pain relief), and discontinued whenever it was inadvisable (e.g. for bradycardia and/or hypotension).

DISCUSSION

Infarct size and reinfarction: Early intravenous atenolol

probably reduced the incidence of completed infarction in patients with threatened infarction (2P< 0.02) and definitely reduced infarct size, as estimated either by ECG or by enzyme measurements, in patients with definite infarcts (2P< 0.001 for each method independently). The reduction in enzymes by early intravenous beta-blockade had already been reported by other workers,[14,16] but the parallel reduction in the ECG estimate of infarct size had not. Unlike Peter et al,[14] we found a reduction in these indices of infarct size both in patients treated very early and in patients treated later than 4 hrs. However, our mean time from pain to entry was only 5 hrs and 88% of patients were admitted within 8 hrs, which should be in time for some benefit to be possible since even at 12 hrs only three-quarters of the ECG evolution of infarction has taken place.[17]

Although the reliability of ECG[18] and that of serum enzymes[19] as strictly quantitative measures of infarct size in experimental infarction have been questioned, both remain useful but indirect indicators of the severity of myocardial damage,[20-23] and reasonable correlations have been demonstrated between them.[13,24] Since we have demonstrated a reduction in infarct size by both indices, it is doubly unlikely that our findings reflect merely methodological artefacts.

In the long-term studies of beta-blockade following discharge from hospital, one of the most marked effects is the reduction in the risk of reinfarction,[25] and we have observed a similar effect during the 10 days of beta-blockade in this study. This, together with the reduction in infarct size, may have been partly responsible for the apparent decrease in intraventricular conduction defects, atrial fibrillation and heart failure - suggesting better left ventricular function - and hence for the decreased use of diuretics and digoxin.

Cardiac arrests and mortality: There is a moderately significant reduction in total mortality at the end of the 10-day treatment period, and although the numbers are too small for subdivision of them to be reliable we did find a difference in early mortality both in patients treated very early (0-4 hrs after

onset of pain) and in patients treated only moderately early
(three-quarters of whom entered 5-8 hrs after onset of pain).
Since patients with cardiac arrest would almost invariably die
if not resuscitated, a pooled analysis of death and/or arrest
might also be appropriate. Such a pool yields 11 vs 25 (2P = 0.01)
affected patients by day 10, and inclusion of reinfarction in this
pool of major events would enhance the apparent protective effect
still further. This difference might be due partly to the
anti-arrhythmic effects[15] of beta-blockade, and partly to their
effects on infarct size. But, overemphasis on combinations of
endpoints can engender misleadingly extreme P-values. Moreover,
no material protection against mortality has been reported in
the aggregate of all other short-term trials of intravenous
treatment,[26] so any true effect on mortality is likely to be
considerably smaller than is suggested by our data.

Side-effects: We observed few dangerous side-effects that
could be attributed to beta-blockade. Although there was
a non-significant excess of sinus arrest, there were no
differences in the numbers with A-V block or pacemaker insertion.
Bradycardia and hypotension were more frequent in the treated
group, but they were usually easily reversible, the use of
atropine and inotropic agents being similar. This does not show
that the risk of treatment inducing one or other of these
conditions is zero, but merely that it is small. For example, one
patient with two previous infarctions developed profound
hypotension (BP unrecordable) immediately following intravenous
atenolol, and was discharged alive only after infusion of high
doses of dopamine, dobutamine and noradrenaline. Although
moderate hypotension and bradycardia are the intended effect of
intravenous beta-blockade, even centres familiar with such
treatment should carefully exclude patients who might be
unsuitable for it, and should be ready to intervene promptly if
serious adverse effects appear.

CONCLUSION
The prevention of full infarction and the limitation of
infarct size have also been seen in other studies of early

intravenous treatment,[14,16,27] and although they have not been
seen in trials of oral treatment this may chiefly be because
of the delay in those trials between administration and full
effect. However, the corresponding reductions in 10-day
reinfarction, cardiac arrest and mortality that we have seen
have not been reported in other randomised trials of intravenous
beta-blockade.[26] Although Hjalmarson et al[28] reported a
reduction in mortality after three months of oral beta-blockade
following initial intravenous treatment, the difference in
mortality was not marked at 10 days and the main effect was
seen only after this period. Late mortality may be affected by
early intravenous treatment, but it is impossible to know
whether the results in Hjalmarson's study were chiefly
produced by the effects of early treatment or by those of
longer-term beta-blockade,[26] as seen in the Norwegian timolol
trial[25] and the Beta-blocker Heart Attack Trial.[29]

Thus, although early intravenous beta-blockade does
consistently appear to reduce infarct size, its effects on
mortality are less certain, especially in general use by a wide
range of centres. An international randomised study (the ISIS
trial) of such treatment is therefore now in progress among
many thousands of patients in 160 different hospitals, and this
should provide a reliable assessment of the net effects of early
intravenous beta-blockade on mortality.

SUMMARY

We report a randomised trial of early intravenous atenolol
(followed by 10 days of oral atenolol) among patients entering
coronary care (i) within 12 hours (mean = 5 hours) of onset of
chest pain suggestive of MI, (ii) not already on beta-blockers,
and (iii) with no clear indication for them (e.g. pain,
hypertension) or against them (e.g. failure, shock or heart
block). Some 20-30% remained eligible, about half of whom
(477 patients) were randomised. The main endpoint was eventual
infarct size, as estimated by enzyme and/or ECG changes. If
definite ECG changes were already present at entry, atenolol
reduced CKMB release by 31% $\pm$ 8% (2P = 0.001), and significantly

enhanced R-wave preservation (2P<0.001). If not, 49% of the
atenolol-allocated patients and 66% of controls subsequently
developed definite infarction (2P<0.02). During the 10-day
treatment period, fewer atenolol-allocated than control patients
died (7 vs 16); suffered cardiac arrest (4 vs 15); or were
recorded as having suffered heart failure (46 vs 56), atrial
fibrillation (12 vs 28), intraventricular conduction defects
(15 vs 28), reinfarction (0 vs 6), or cardiogenic shock (1 vs 4).
Of the 10-day survivors, 12.2% of atenolol-allocated and 12.4%
of controls are known to have died subsequently.

ACKNOWLEDGEMENTS

We thank Dr. J. D. Harry, Mrs. L. Booth, Mrs. P. Lowery,
ICI; the house physicians, the nursing staff of both CCUs and
the physicians of both hospitals for their assistance.

This study was supported by the British Heart Foundation and
ICI Pharmaceuticals.

Gale Mead and Jini Hetherington prepared the typescript.

REFERENCES

1. Sobel BE, Bresnahan GF, Shell WE, Yoder RD: Estimation of
   infarct size in man and its relation to prognosis.
   Circulation (46): 640-648, 1972.

2. Schlant RC, Foreman S, Stamler J, Canner PL: The natural
   history of coronary heart disease: prognostic factors after
   recovery from myocardial infarction in 2789 men. The 5-year
   findings of the Coronary Drug Project. Circulation (66):
   401-414, 1982.

3. Miura M, Thomas R, Ganz W, Sokol T, Shell WE, Toshimitsu T,
   Chin Kwan A, Singh BN: The effect of delay in propranolol
   administration on reduction of myocardial infarct size after
   experimental coronary artery occlusion in dogs. Circulation
   (59): 1148-1157, 1979.

4. Thompson PC, Jones AS, Noon D, Katavatis V: A randomised trial
   of oral beta-blockade during myocardial infarction: lack of
   effect on enzymatic indices of myocardial necrosis.
   Aust NZ Med J (9): 757 (abstr), 1979.

5. Roland JM, Wilcox RG, Banks DC, Edwards B, Fentem PH,
   Hampton JR: Effect of beta-blockers on arrhythmias during six
   weeks after suspected myocardial infarction. Br med J (ii):
   518-521, 1979.

6. Balcon R, Jewitt DE, Davis JPH, Oram SA: A controlled trial of propranolol in acute myocardial infarction. Lancet (ii): 917-920, 1966.

7. Clausen J, Felsby M, Schonan Jorgensen F, Lyager Neilsen B, Roin J, Strange B: Absence of prophylactic effect of propranolol in myocardial infarction. Lancet (ii): 820-824, 1966.

8. Wilcox RG, Roland JM, Banks DC, Hampton JR, Mitchell JRA: Randomised trial comparing propranolol with atenolol in immediate treatment of suspected myocardial infarction. Br med J (280): 885-888, 1980.

9. Rutherford JD, Singh BN, Ambler PK, Norris RM: Plasma propranolol concentration in patients with angina and acute myocardial infarction. Clin Exp Pharmacol Physiol (3): 297-304, 1976.

10. Yusuf S: Beta adrenergic blockade in acute myocardial infarction. D.Phil thesis: University of Oxford, 1980.

11. Yusuf S, Peto R, Bennett D, Sleight P, Ramsdale R, Furse L, Bray C: Early intravenous atenolol treatment in suspected acute myocardial infarction. Lancet (ii): 273-276, 1980.

12. Norris RM, Whitlock RML, Barratt-Boyes C, Small CW: Clinical measurement of myocardial infarct size: modification of a method for the estimation of creatinine phosphokinase release after myocardial infarction. Circulation (51): 614-620, 1975.

13. Yusuf S, Lopez R, Maddison A, Maw P, Ray N, McMillan S, Sleight P: Value of electrocardiogram in predicting and estimating infarct size in man. Br Heart J (42): 286-293, 1979.

14. Peter T, Norris RM, Clarke ED, Heng MK, Singh BN, Williams B, Howell DR, Ambler PK: Reduction of enzyme levels by propranolol after acute myocardial infarction. Circulation (57): 1091-1095, 1978.

15. Rossi PRF, Yusuf S, Ramsdale D, Furse LY, Sleight P: Reduction of ventricular arrhythmias by early intravenous atenolol in suspected acute myocardial infarction. Br med J (in press), 1983.

16. Jurgensen HJ, Frederiksen J, Hansen DA, Pedersen-Bjergaard O: Limitation of myocardial infarct size in patients less than 60 years treated with alprenolol. Br Heart J (45): 583-588, 1981.

17. Yusuf S, Lopez R, Maddison A, Sleight P: Variability of electrocardiographic and enzyme evolution of myocardial infarction in man. Br Heart J (45): 271-280, 1981.

18. Holland RP, Arnsdorf MR: Solid angle theory and the electrocardiogram: physiologic and quantitative interpretations. Progr Cardiovasc Dis (XIX(6)): 430-457, 1977.

19. Roe CR, Cobb FR, Starmer CF: The relationship between enzymatic and histologic estimates of the extent of myocardial infarction in conscious dogs with permanent coronary occlusion. Circulation (55): 438-449, 1977.

20. Bleifeld WH, Hanrath P, Mathey D: Serial CPK determinations for evaluation of size and development of acute myocardial infarction. Circulation (53) Suppl I: 108, 1976.

21. Muller JE, Maroko PR, Braunwald E: Praecordial electrocardiographic mapping. Circulation (57): 1-18, 1978.

22. Palmeri ST, Harrison DG, Cobb FR, Morris KG, Harrell FE, Ideker RE, Selvester RH, Wagner GS: A QRS scoring system for assessing left ventricular function after myocardial infarction. New Engl J Med (306): 4-9, 1982.

23. Grande P, Hansen, BF, Christiansen C, Naestoft J: Estimation of acute myocardial infarct size in man by serum CK-MB measurements. Circulation (66): 756-763, 1982.

24. Henning H, Hardarson H, Francis G, O'Rourke AR, Ryan W, Ross J Jr: Approach to the estimation of myocardial infarct size by analysis of praecordial ST segment and R wave maps. Amer J Cardiol (41): 1-7, 1978.

25. The Norwegian Multicentre Study Group: Timolol-induced reduction in mortality and reinfarction in patients surviving acute myocardial infarction. New Engl J Med (304): 801-807, 1981.

26. Editorial: Long-term and short-term beta-blockade after myocardial infarction. Lancet (i): 1159-1161, 1982.

27. Norris RM, Clarke ED, Sammel NL, Smith WM: Protective effect of propranolol in threatened myocardial infarction. Lancet (ii): 907-909, 1978.

28. Hjalmarson A, Herlitz J, Malek I, Ryden L, Vedin A, Waldenstrom A, Wedel H, Elmfeldt D, Holmberg S, Nyberg G, Swedberg K, Waagstein F, Waldenstrom J, Wilhelmsen L: Effect on mortality of metoprolol in acute myocardial infarction. Lancet (ii): 823-827, 1981.

29. Beta-blocker Heart Attack Study Group. The beta-blocker heart attack trial. JAMA (246): 2073-2074. 1981.

17

Calcium Channel Blockers and Limitation of Myocardial Infarction Size

Zoltan G. Turi, M.D.

Initial great enthusiasm for the use of calcium channel blocking agents in acute myocardial infarction (AMI) stems from the work of Oliva (1) in which 40% of patients catheterized immediately after onset of symptoms could be demonstrated to have restoration of flow through a previously occluded coronary vessel following the selective intracoronary injection of nitroglycerin. These findings coincided with those of Maseri (2) that some patients with reversible coronary vasospasm would eventually develop myocardial infarction in the same vascular distribution. Thus, drugs with potent coronary spasmolytic effect, such as calcium channel blocking agents, might be highly effective in restoring flow to infarcting areas of myocardium.

Unfortunately, subsequent data, derived from routine intracoronary nitroglycerin infusion that precedes the administration of thrombolytic therapy, have demonstrated that only 5-10% of obstructed coronary arteries can be re-opened with a vasodilator (3). Nevertheless, calcium channel blocking agents may exert a variety of beneficial clinical effects in salvaging ischemic myocardium because of their potent inhibition of calcium ion flux across cell membranes in myocardial cells and vascular smooth muscle (Table I).

Table I

Mechanisms for Myocardial Preservation
with Calcium Channel Blocking Agents

1. Increase myocardial oxygen supply
    a. Prevent coronary artery spasm
    b. Improve collateral blood flow
2. Decrease myocardial oxygen demand
    a. Decrease afterload
    b. Decrease contractility
    c. Decrease heart rate
3. Prevent intracellular calcium overload
4. Alter myocardial energy metabolism

For the minority of patients in whom coronary obstruction is due to coronary vasoconstriction alone, calcium channel blocking agents will maximize the myocardial oxygen supply:demand ratio by relieving or preventing coronary vasospasm.

In patients with severe fixed atherosclerotic disease or acute thrombus formation (even if spasm has been the original precipitating event with stasis and thrombosis occurring as a secondary phenomenon) calcium channel blocking agents may improve myocardial oxygen supply:demand either by improving collateral blood flow to the ischemic zone or by substantially decreasing myocardial oxygen demand. The clinical effects on heart rate, blood pressure and some indices of contractility differ markedly among these drugs, primarily because of baroreceptor mediated reflex sympathetic activity due to peripheral vasodilatation (Table II).

Table II
Effects of Ca^{++} Channel Blockers
on Myocardial Oxygen Supply and Demand

Demand

	Nifedipine	Verapamil	Diltiazem
Blood Pressure	↓↓	↓	↓
Heart Rate	↑	±	↓
Contractility	↑	±↓	O
Preload	O	O	O

Supply

	Nifedipine	Verapamil	Diltiazem
Coronary Blood Flow	↑	↑	↑

(Adapted from Stone PH: Use of calcium channel blocking agents to salvage ischemic myocardium (4). By permission.)

In addition, calcium channel blocking agents, by preventing calcium influx during ischemia, prevent the harmful effects of calcium overload which may accelerate cell death: namely the accumulation of calcium in the mitochondria, which leads to the depletion of intracellular ATP and resultant inability to maintain efficient energy requiring intracellular ion transport (5). An elegant experiment by Clark (6) demonstrates the preservation of contractility and reduction of diastolic stiffness associated with the use of nifedipine during ischemia (Figure 1).

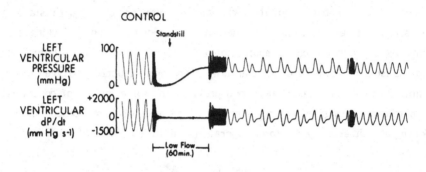

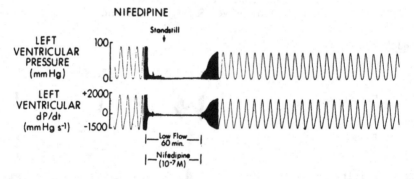

(Figure 1. Effect of nifedipine on recovery from ischemia by the isolated perfused rabbit heart. From Clark RE: Nifedipine: A myocardial protective agent (6). By permission)

A fourth beneficial mechanism may be changes in energy metabolism induced by calcium channel blockade unrelated to the hemodynamic effects of these agents; including a shift to carbohydrate metabolism because of drug-induced inhibition of endogenous lipolysis (7). A fifth beneficial effect in AMI, seen with verapamil, is a prevention of the fall of the ventricular fibrillation threshold that is associated with both acute ischemia and reperfusion (8).

In the experimental animal model, verapamil and nifedipine have been shown to decrease infarct size (9,10) and diltiazem has been demonstrated to increase coronary blood flow to epicardial and endocardial ischemic areas without substantial reduction in infarct size (11). An animal study of particular relevance is that of Selwyn (12) demonstrating the dose-related threshold effect of nifedipine after coronary occlusion. With administration of 1 µg/kg nifedipine a decrease in infarct size may be demonstrated; a 13 µg/kg infusion resulted in excessive hypotension with reflex tachycardia and an increase in regional ischemia and infarct size.

<u>Human Studies with Calcium Channel Blocking Agents</u>

Small non-blinded non-randomized trials with nifedipine were performed demonstrating relative safety of administration of 10 mg to 20 mg po during acute myocardial infarction (13,14). All investigators noted a fall in blood pressure; this appears to parallel decreases in left ventricular filling pressure (15).

A preliminary report of a randomized and placebo-controlled prospective trial of 54 patients who were administered intravenous verapamil 5 to 10 mg per hour at a mean of 8 hours after the onset of symptoms appeared to demonstrate a reduction in both peak creatine kinase as well as infarct size as measured by extrapolation from serum enzyme curves. Except for a 10 mmHg decrease in systemic arterial pressure, no major hemodynamic effect was observed in this group of patients, who had a pulmonary arterial wedge pressure of less than 15 mmHg at the onset of treatment (16).

A large randomized, double-blind and placebo controlled study has recently been completed which investigated the role of nifedipine in patients with AMI. The Nifedipine in Angina and Myocardial Infarction Study (NAMIS) screened 3,114 patients admitted to the coronary care units at participating intitutions (17). Eligible patients included those who had greater than 45 minutes of chest pain, could receive the treatment assignment less than 6 hours after onset of symptoms, and demonstrated new or presumably new ST segment elevation or depression of at least 0.1 mV or demonstrated new Q waves. One hundred and eighty one patients were randomized, the remainder were excluded either because of protocol exclusion or because they refused consent. The purpose of the study was to determine if therapy with nifedipine (20 mg po every 4 hours) could prevent progression from a threatened to acute myocardial infarction and, secondly, to demonstrate if nifedipine limits infarct size in patients who progress to infarction or who are already infarcting at the time of randomization.

Eighty-two patients were treated with placebo and 89 with nifedipine; an additional 10 patients were randomized who were found to be ineligible either for not having met ECG criteria or because they were classified as "threatened" myocardial infarction when in fact enzymes drawn at the time of randomization demonstrated an already evolving infarction.

There was no difference between the placebo and nifedipine treated patients in either progression to infarction in those who were classified as "threatened" MI nor was there a difference in infarct size index in those patients who infarcted; pain relief was faster in nifedipine treated patients (Table III).

Table III

Nifedipine (N) vs. Placebo (P) in NAMIS

	N	P	p
Infarct incidence	73%	75%	NS
Infarct size index (CK)	15.2 ±1.4	15.1 ±1.2	NS
Mortality - 2 weeks	8%	0%	<.05
Mortality - 6 months	11%	7%	NS

(From Muller J et al:Nifedipine therapy for threatened and acute myocardial infarction (17). By permission of the American Heart Association, Inc.)

Mortality in the group treated with nifedipine was greater than that of the placebo group, although this result reached statistical significance only if a retrospectively selected two week endpoint was chosen and only if the 10 patients initially randomized but subsequently found ineligible were excluded from the overall analysis. No statistically significant difference was seen in 6 month mortality between treated and nontreated groups. Of particular note is the unusual finding of zero deaths in the placebo group; this contrast with a 4.8% mortality among eligible non-randomized patients, none of whom was treated with calcium channel blockade. Finally, when the 10 randomized, but subsequently found to be ineligible, patients are included in the statistical analysis there was no statistically significant difference in either 2 week or 6 month mortality.

No significant differences were noted in untoward effects in the treated and untreated groups: specifically there was no difference in incidence of vasodilator side effects (headache, drop in systolic arterial pressure to < 80 mmmHg), nausea or vomiting. In addition, although there was a trend suggesting higher mortality in the nifedipine treated group, this could not be explained by any increase in infarct size.

Given the trial design and numbers of patients enrolled, there was an 80% probability that a reduction of infarct size of 30% or greater would have been detected. Thus, administration of nifedipine a mean of 5.2 ± 2.5 hours after the onset of chest pain appeared to have no beneficial effect on myocardial infarct size and did not prevent progression of "threatened" to acute myocardial infarction. The lack of clearly demonstrable beneficial effect on infarct size and suggestion of a greater mortality with the use of this vasodilator in the early post infarction period (first 5 hours) suggest that the routine use of nifedipine immediately after myocardial infarction should await further studies.

Early results from several other trials with calcium channel blocking agents, such as the Danish Multicenter Group study of verapamil (18) have failed to demonstrate clear cut benefit when calcium channel blockade has been administered in the early post-infarction period. Whether this is due to late administration, the need to define the therapeutic/toxic range more accurately (as suggested by Selwyn's data[12]) or possibly species specificity of the beneficial effects seen with calcium channel blocker use in animals is unclear.

It is clear from animal laboratory experimental data and strongly suggested by human drug trials that interventions to limit myocardial infarct size should take place in the early hours post infarction (19,20). While there is some data that suggest benefit up to 18 hours after MI (21), this may be related not to preservation of jeopardized myocardium but to mechanisms such as prevention of infarct extension. Clearly early intervention, preferably within 3 to 4 hours of onset of symptoms, is desirable, both to salvage tissue as well as to intervene during the exponentially rising mortality phase in the post myocardial infarction patient.

The recently released results of the propranolol wing of the Multicenter Investigation of the Limitation of Infarct Size (MILIS) study (22) failed to show improvement in mortality or decrease in infarct size when propranolol (0.1 mg/kg i.v. followed by oral therapy for 9 days) was administered a mean of 8.9 hours after onset of symptoms. These results contrast with those of Yusuf (23) and Peter (24) whose administration was earlier: 5 and <4 hours for i.v. atenolol and propranolol respectively. Because of substantial differences in study design, timing of the intervention was probably not the sole cause of the divergent results.

Finally, the results of the BHAT and Timolol trials (25,26) clearly demonstrate improvement in mortality with late (5-21 days and 7-28 days respectively) oral administration of β-blockade. The approximately 25% of patients who do not tolerate β-blockade in this time window may be candidates for calcium channel blocking agents. This, as well as the potential benefit of combined β-blockade and calcium blockade, is under active investigation in this country and abroad.

REFERENCES

1. Oliva PB, Breckinridge JC: Arteriographic evidence of coronary arterial spasm in acute myocardial infarction. Circulation (56):366-374, 1977.

2. Maseri A, L'Abbate A, Baroldi G, Chierchia S, Marzilli M, Ballestra AM, Severi S, Parodi O, Biagini A, Distante A, Pesola A: Coronary vasospasm as a possible cause of myocardial infarction: A conclusion derived from the study of "preinfarction" angina. New Engl J Med (299):1271-1277, 1978.

3. Ganz W, Buchbinder N, Marcus H, Mondkar A, Maddahi J, Charuzi Y, O'Connor L, Shell W, Fishbein MC, Kass R, Mujamoto A, Swan HJC: Intracoronary thrombolysis in evolving myocardial infarction. Am Heart J (101):4-13, 1981.

4. Stone PH:Use of calcium channel blocking agents to salvage ischemic myocardium. In: Hoffman BF, ed. Calcium antagonists: The state of the art and role in cardiovascular disease. Symposia on Fromtiers of Pharmacology (2): 209-223, 1983.

5. Fleckenstein A: Specific inhibitors and promoters of calcium action in the excitation contraction coupling of heart muscle and their role in the prevention of production of myocardial lesions. In: Harris P, Opie L, eds. Calcium and the heart. Academic Press, New York, 1971, pp 135-188.

6. Clark RE, Christlieb IY, Henry PD, Fischer AE, Nora JD, Williamson JR, Sobel BE: Nifedipine: A myocardial protective agent. Am J Cardiol (44):825-831, 1979.

7. Verdouw PD, ten Cate FJ, Hartog M, Scheffer MG, Stam H: Intracoronary infusion of small doses of nifedipine lowers regional myocardial O_2-consumption without altering regional myocardial function. Basic Res Cardiol (77):26-33, 1982.

8. Brooks WW, Verrier RL, Lown B: Protective effect of verapamil on vulnerability to ventricular fibrillation during myocardial ischaemia and reperfusion. Cardiovasc Res (14):295-302, 1980.

9. Henry PD, Shuchleib R, Borda LJ, Roberts R, Williamson JR, Sobel BE: Effects of nifedipine on myocardial perfusion and ischemic injury in dogs. Circ Res (43):372-380, 1978.

10. DeBoer LWV, Strauss HW, Kloner RA, Rude RE, Davis RF, Maroko PR, Braunwald E: Autoradiographic method of measuring the ischemic myocardium at risk: effects of verapamil on infarct size after experimental coronary artery occlusion. Proc Natl Acad Sci USA (77):6119-6123, 1980.

11. Nakamura M, Kajwaya Y, Yamada A, et al: Effects of diltiazem, a new antianginal drug on myocardial blood flow following experimental coronary occlusion. In: Winbury MM, Abiko Y, eds. Ischemic Myocardium and Antianginal Drugs. Raven Press, New York, 1979, pp 129-142.

12. Selwyn AP, Welman E, Fox K, Harlock P, Pratt T, Klein M: The effects of nifedipine on acute experimental myocardial ischemia and infarction in dogs. Circ Res (44):16-23, 1979.

13. Bussmann WD, Schofer H, Kaltenbach M: Die hamodynamische Wirkung von Nifedipine bei akutem Herzinfarkt. Herz/Kreislauf (9)(3):140-147, 1977.

14. Deaisieux J-C, et al: Hemodynamic effects of a single oral dose of nifedipine following acute myocardial infarction. Chest (78):574, 1980.

15. Roberts R, Jaffe AS, Henry PD, Sobel BE: Nifedipine and acute myocardial infarction. Herz (6):90-97, 1981.

16. Bussman WD, Seher W, Grungras M, Klepzig H: Reduktioin der Ck-und CKMB-Infarktgrosse durch intravenose Gabe von Verapamil. Zeitschrift fur Kardiologie (71):164, 1982.

17. Muller J, Morrison J, Stone P, Rude R, Rosner B, Roberts R, Pearle D, Turi Z, Schneider J, Serfas D, Hennekens C, Braunwald E: Nifedipine therapy for threatened and acute myocardial infarction: A randomized double blind comparison. Circulation (68)(Suppl II):III-120, 1983.

18. Danish Multicenter Group. Verapamil in acute myocardial infarction. Clin Exp Pharm Physiol (6):89,1982.

19. Hillis LD, Fishbein MC, Braunwald E, Maroko PR: The influence of the time interval between coronary artery occlusion and the administration of hyaluronidase on salvage of ischemic myocardium in dogs. Circ Res (41):26-31, 1977.

20. Miura M, Thomas R, Ganz W, Sokol T, Shell WE, Toshimitsu T, Kwan AC, Singh BN: The effect of delay in propranolol administration on reduction of myocardial infarct size after experimental coronary artery occlusion in dogs. Circulation (59):1148-1157, 1979.

21. Reduto LA, Freund GC, Gaeta JM: Coronary artery reperfusion in acute myocardial infarction: Beneficial effects of intracoronary streptokinase on left ventricular salvage and performance. Am Heart J (102):1168, 1981.

22. Muller J, Roberts R, Stone P, Rude R, Raabe D, Gold H, Jaffe A, Strauss W, Turi Z, Hartwell T, Poole K, Passamani E, Willerson J, Sobel B, Braunwald E, and MILIS Group:Failure of propranolol administration to limit infarct size in patients with acute myocardial infarction. Circulation (68) (Suppl III):III-294, 1983.

23. Yusuf S, Sleight P, Rossi P, Ramsdale D, Peto R, Furze L, Sterry H, Pearson M, Motwani R, Parish S, Gray R, Bennett D, Bray C: Reduction in infarct size, arrhythmias and chest pain by early intravenous beta blockade in suspected acute myocardial infarction. Circulation (67)(Suppl I):I-32-I-41, 1983.

24. Peter T, Norris RM, Clarke ED, Heng MK, Singh BN, Williams B, Howell DR, Ambler PK: Reduction of Enzyme Levels by Propranolol After Acute Myocardial Infarction. Circulation (57):1091-1095, 1978.

25. Norwegian Multicenter Study Group: Timolol-induced reduction in mortality and reinfarction in patients surviving acute myocardial infarction. N Eng J Med (304):801, 1981.

26. β-Blocker Heart Attack Trial Research Group: A randomized trial of propranolol in patients with acute myocardial infarction: I. Mortality results. JAMA (247):1707-1714.

18

STEROID TREATMENT OF ACUTE MYOCARDIAL INFARCTION: SOME
IMPLICATIONS FOR CLINICAL TRIALS IN GENERAL

P.L. DERN, M.D.

1. INTRODUCTION

Glucocorticoid studies of infarct size illustrate features
of more general interest for clinical trials. A point of note
is the close relationship of studies in animals to those in
humans.

2. SOME EXPERIMENTAL BACKGROUND

Glucocorticoids reduced infarct size when given up to 6
hours after coronary ligation in animals.[1] Treatment after
7 hours with one or two doses decreased or had no effect on
infarct size in men.[2,3] Multiple doses in a patient was
associated with delayed healing and aneurysm formation.[4]
Dogs with experimental myocardial infarction showed delayed
healing of infarcts after one intravenous and one intramuscular
dose of glucocorticoids given in a 6 hour interval after onset
of ischemia.[5] Multiple doses in humans increased arrhythmia
rates and increased infarct size.[3]

3. SPECIFICATION OF PROBLEMS

3.1. Baseline subgroup interaction with treatment

Preliminary studies may suggest strongly that a particular
baseline characteristic is likely to influence response to
treatment in a future clinical trial. Instead of pooling
responses over all levels of the key variable the hope is
that examination of the treatment effect within two or more
levels will increase the precision of the estimate. This is
not usually done in the initial clinical trials of drugs
for mortality endpoints in part because no one variable may

be of dominant interest. Another difficulty is that separate
clinical trials must be carried out within each level of the
factor.

3.2. <u>Multiple endpoints</u>

Multiple endpoints are usually dealt with by specifying
one, say total mortality, in a primary hypothesis upon
which the sample size requirements of the trial are then
calculated. Secondary hypotheses are then constructed to
use the other endpoints. Statistical methods and inferences
are standard ones. This traditional use of endpoints may
not conform to the sequence of events in the disease under
study and different approaches can be made to supplement
the traditional ones. For example, infarct size might be
considered an indication of a preliminary state from which
other endpoints develop.

4. SUMMARY

Special problems and opportunities arise when the
preliminary findings of studies suggest key variables
and endpoints for examination in clinical trials.

REFERENCES

1. Libby P, Maroko PR, Bloor CH, Sobel BE, Braunwald E:
   Reduction of experimental myocardial infarct size by
   corticosteroid administration. J Clin Invest. 52: 599-606,
   1973.

2. Morrison J, Reduto L, Pizzarello R, Geller K, Maley T,
   Gullota S: Modification of myocardial injury in man by
   corticosteroid administration. Circulation 51: I200-203,
   1976.

3. Roberts R, de Melli V, Sobel BE: Deleterious effects of
   methylprednisolone in patients with myocardial infarction.
   Circulation 53: I204-206, 1976.

4. Bulkley BH, Roberts WC: Steroid therapy during acute
   myocardial infarction. Am J Med 56: 244-250, 1974.

5. Green RM, Cohen J, DeWeese JA: Short-term use of
   corticoids after experimental myocardial infarction: effects
   on ventricular function and infarct healing. Circulation
   50: I101-103, 1974.

19

EVALUATION OF INOTROPIC THERAPY

Dr. Raymond Lipicky

It makes sense to use inotropic intervention, if indeed the
circulation is inadequate and may for example in myocardial
infarction extend that infarct. Caution is required since there are
hypotheses that are reasonably supported by data that suggest that high
intracellular calcium concentrations stimulate mitochondria to respond
faster, to respire faster and that these in turn raise calcium
concentration further and that eventually because of raised intracellular
calcium concentration, the cell dies a hypoxic death. That really raises
a kind of caution in that any inotropic intervention in all probability
will deal at some phase in its action by raising intracellular calcium
concentrations and that indeed one would have to more seriously consider
the possibility that inotropic intervention may in fact be deleterious
especially if some cells are marginal. If one is measuring hemodynamic
effects grossly in the entire circulatory system, these marginal cells in
fact might be injured quite significantly and lead to a real undetected
deleterious effect. I would like to discuss what kinds of things one might
accept from an inotropic intervention.

If one uses an anesthetized dog model to determine a dose response
relationship with contractile force as the end point, it is quite
reasonable to expect the measurement if contractile force can be a dose
related event and one can see the shape of the dose response curve. One
can also measure systole and diastolic blood pressures and peripheral
resistance and see an effect of the drug on peripheral resistance. If the
effects on peripheral vasculature seem to come in somewhere different from
where the effects of the ionotropic intervention and there is very little
in the way of direct heart rate effect (except when blood pressure begins
to fall) than this might be a reasonable drug to begin exploring in man
with respect to its inotropic effects. If one were to look for inotropic
effects in man, it is also reasonable to probably choose as the primary

patient material, patients with congestive heart failure. It is probably
also reasonable to choose patients with relatively severe congestive heart
failure since it is most likely in that circumstance that one can see the
most reasonable drug changes. If one is going to do that, it is also
reasonable to require (and I think we do), that some invasive methods be
used to measure cardiac index directly with a calculation of the peripheral
resistance and filling pressures to see that the pressures and cardiac
output are changed in appropriate directions.

In the development of amrinone in fact, 67% of the patients with class
IV congestive heart failure that constituted the base of knowledge about
that drug, and the average cardiac index in those patients was 1.84 and the
average wedge pressure was about 27. If one studies such a population and
in fact measures an increase in cardiac index, a decrease in pulmonary
wedge pressure, with little change in the heart rate or mean arterial
pressure, it is not unreasonable to say that this kind of data would
absolutely confirm that the drug has a positive inotropic effect in man.
The number of patients that were involved in actually presenting that
confirmation were only 7, and it was also possible to see that there was
not much of an effect on myocardial oxygen uptake or any indirect
measurement such as arterial lactate differences.

Having confirmed that like in another mammalian system, the drug has a
positive inotropic effect, it would be reasonable then to pursue the
problem of how does this effect relate to dose since after all the only
variable that is controllable is what dose one administers and that indeed
is a reasonable variable to define. If one is confronted with the problem
of making basic measurements in people with congestive heart failure who
are very sick, what frequently happens, is that all measurements can't be
made in all patients at all doses and at the right times and that there is
lots of missing information. So that if one attempts to deal with the data
in any statistical form, it really can't be done. What can one do? Well,
what was done here was to find out of 116 patients that were studied, 13
that had received only bolus injections of amrinone but indeed had received
more than 1 bolus injection and that each injection was at a different dose
and in whom there was some kind of serial measurement of parameters with
time after the dose. Not all patients had measurements at all times; not
all patients had every dose; nonetheless one can see that a bolus of 3
mg/kg produces a bigger effect than 0.5 mg/kg. In fact there appears to be

a dose related peak effect and that on the whole the duration of effect was also dose dependent. All logical conclusions were supported by the data. Moreover, if one takes those same 13 patients and simply looks at the peak change from baseline (in patients who had more than one dose) that indeed there is some kind of a shape that goes on and one could actually even use that data and even put it into models. This is dose response modeling. The particular line that is drawn is best done by a empirical quadratic equation. This approach suggests that there is an inflection that best fits the data and that that inflection is somewhere in the 0.4 to 0.5 mg/kg range and that there is a slope to the line. What it doesn't define is whether or not the slope turns over. In only 13 patients the reliability of the data must be questioned.

If one collects blood samples from these patients, one indeed sees that there is a general relationship to blood level. One way of testing the hypothesis that that sample of 13 in fact has some predictive value is to now say, let's look at all measurements from every single patient that had a measurement at any dose that we can define in some fashion, either in people who had bolus injections or infusions or combination of bolus injection and infusions. Indeed, what you see is there were hypothetically 3 patients who had this dose and had a measurement of cardiac index. There were 41 patients that had this dose and had a measurement of cardiac index. There were 19 that had this dose and a measurement of cardiac index, so there aren't equal numbers of people all over, but indeed there is a dose related effect on cardiac index and that the relationship begins somewhere in the neighborhood of 0.5 mg/kg and extends out to somewhere in the neighborhood of 6.0 or higher. If one sees that the pulmonary-capillary wedge pressure is similarly defined in uneven numbers of patients, and has a relationship to dose and bears the same relationship to dose as does the cardiac index and that indeed the peripheral vascular resistance and mean arterial pressure are related to dose and that it does not really begin to change significantly until at a dose beyond where there is clear manifestation of inotropic activity, then one gets a reasonable feeling for a dose response relationship that certainly satisfies at least my need to see that there is a positive inotropic effect in man and that the effect is dose related and that it is predictable.

To conclude that there is a positive inotropic effect, that is probably all the data that one needs. Knowing that a positive inotropic effect is there, probably is not sufficient information however. It would have been nice in those particular patients had some consequence of the positive inotropic effect been measured. Could it have been as simple as urinary output? Some kind of quantitation of rales, cardiac size on x-ray which would then give one a feeling that indeed the positive inotropic effect led somewhere. I think that if one didn't have that evidence knowing that a positive inotropic effect was present would be insufficent in that you don't know what it means. Within the context of myocardial infarction, you clearly need to be very suspicious that it may have an adverse effect and in all probability if one were thinking about an inotropic intervention in acute myocardial infarction, the end point that one would really have to be seriously interested in would be cardiac mortality.

20

PANEL ON PHARMACEUTICAL INTERVENTIONS TO REDUCE INFARCT SIZE (continued)

Moderator: Dr. Joel Morganroth

Dr. Morganroth: I have always been concerned about the use of beta
blocker therapy in patients with acute phase of myocardial infarction since
if coronary spasm is present beta blockade may be deleterious. I wonder if
this is the reason the acute beta blocker trials seem to be close to the no
significance line. I wonder if you would comment on your concern, Dr.
Sleight, as a clinician in giving beta blocker therapy in this setting and
also comment on whether an ultra short-acting beta blocker might be safer or
more useful?

Dr. Sleight: I think there is no doubt that spasm exists, but I don't find
it all that common in the sort of patients we look at in our unit. I was
interested also in Dr. Turi's nifedipine trial in that didn't really show
that spasm was frequent especially if nifedipine was a useful agent. That
didn't seem to be as beneficial as one might have expected it to be either,
so although spasm occurs, I think it is not terribly common in the ordinary
run of acute myocardial infarction. The second question was about whether it
was better to use a shorter acting beta blocker, I think in many ways it
might be attractive if you had an ultra short-acting beta blocker, at least
if you had an adverse effect, you could be over it quicker. Having said
that, if you want to do a trial, then there is great beauty in choosing a
drug which has a long-lasting effect, because even if the house-man gets cold
feet because the blood pressure is 95, the patient has the treatment and it
sticks there for 24 hours. That turned out to be a useful effect.

Dr. Temple: Dr. Sleight, do patients regularly get nitroglycerine for
continued pain in your study?

Dr Sleight: Yes, they would get whatever additional treatment was
thought clinically indicated.

Dr. Temple: It seems possible to me that anybody who didn't have a spasm component and who therefore had persistent pain or even worse pain, might very well respond to that kind of treatment and therefore one wouldn't notice very much.

Dr. Sleight: Well surely, but the thing that struck me when we analyzed it was that if we took two people with ST elevation that 99.9 % of them actually developed a definite infarction. I say there is one patient who made the difference from 100% who had what seemed in retrospect to be Prinzmetal's angina.

Dr. Morganroth: Are you suggesting Dr. Temple that a stronger study design would be to have no therapy for one of the aims?

Dr. Temple: All I meant was that if there are in other populations more people presenting with spasm, and I don't know why there should be, it may be that the fact that nitroglycerine is regularly given nowadays if pain persists might be masking those people. There is every reason to think spasm would respond to nitrates.

Dr. Turi: Our primary hypothesis was that 40% or so of AMI patients have spasm, but that doesn't seem to be holding up in any of the studies. It seems to be more in the 5-10% range. I think Dr. Temple is correct both on the basis of dog laboratory data and some human experimentation that spasm is certainly not helped by beta blockade, coronary resistance rises, coronary flow decreases, so I don't think there is a clean answer to that particular question but at least the incidence doesn't seem to be very high.

Dr. Henis: Dr. Lipicky, couldn't you have gotten all the same data if amrinone weren't simply a balanced vasodilator. I know there has been some controversy about that.

Dr. Lipicky: I think you could with the singular exception that in the very early part of the dose response relationship (where it clearly separates itself out) what dose you need to significantly affect the periphery in relationship to what dose you need to effect the myocardium is important. Clearly the overall action is a combination of the two. Whether or not the inotropic intervention plays a role I think is shown on the early phases of the dose response relationship.

Dr. Sleight: I know some data from St. Thomas' Hospital which I have seen presented and also seen the manuscript that showed in heart failure patients as compared in to normal man, that indeed there is an inotropic effect that you could demonstrate before you got a vasodilator effect. But in heart failure patients he could not discriminate between the vasodilator effect and the inotropic effect and so he did not find it to have in heart failure patients in contrast to this and I think it was actually a more rigorously examined study. He did not find any inotropic effects. I would still like to keep an open mind.

Dr. Temple: I may mis-remember, but this question was discussed by Dr. Jay Cohn at one of these sessions last year, and even if you take a pure vasodilator like nitroprusside, the initial response is not a fall in blood pressure, presumably because you can compensate for a certain amount of vasodilation without any dramatic heart rate increase and you don't see a fall in blood pressure either. They are not as different as you might think. Although I must say, I think other evidence in isolated tissues, etc., makes it awfully likely that this is in fact behaving as an inotropic agent.

Dr. Sleight: I think there is no doubt that it does so in normal tissue in normal dogs and normal man, but I think it is much harder to show in heart failure patients.

Dr. Ruberio: Dr. Turi, it has been shown England that to give nifedipine into an experimental setting, that a small dose decreased myocardial infarction and a bigger dose increased myocardial infarction. So I would like to ask you what was the rationale for choosing 20 mg 6 times a day, for nifedipine in your patient population?

Dr. Turi: I think I mentioned that Dr. Sullivan demonstrated that 1 ug/kg of nifedipine salvaged myocardium and a 13 fold larger dose, (13 ug/kg) actually resulted in an increase in necrosis. That was the dose that was necessary a 13 fold increase to decrease the blood pressure by 30%. In specific answer to your question regarding why we chose this large a dose, at the time that this study was started and in fact throughout the study, we were rather impressed by the evidence that the primary benefit that we might obtain from calcium channel blockade would be the spasmolytic effect. I listed 4 different potential beneficial effects, many of them having to do with preserving ischemic myocardium. The one that we were most impressed with and the one for which we had the greatest hope was the spasmolytic effect, the potential benefit of being able to reverse coronary spasm and since that was the end point and the mechanism of action we were shooting for. We wanted to get the maximal possible chance of a spasmolytic effect which we felt would require a higher dose. In retrospect, there are several things to consider. One of them is that other studies that have started with lower dosage forms and worked their way up following the blood pressure have not seen this possibly significant effect that we saw with regard to mortality and probably if we had this study to do all over again, we would not have started with such a high dose.

<u>Dr. Ruberio:</u>   What were the hemodynamic effects that you accomplished?

<u>Dr. Turi:</u> Actually, there was a non-statistically significant lowering of blood pressure in the nifedipine group versus the placebo group. If one analyzes the number of patients who developed significant hypotension that is blood pressure, less than 85 mm/Hg, the difference between the nifedipine group and placebo group was not significant. There was a slight trend, but it was not significant. Of the 7 patients who died in the treated group, only 2 of them became clearly hypotensive, so although one of the postulates for why there might have been an excess of deaths was the induction of hypotension in these patients. It really does not seem to bear out when one tries to analyze the data.

<u>Dr. Ruberio:</u>   Dr. Sleight, you beautifully documented the beneficial effects of altenolol after myocardial infarction. Dr. Turi presented the data at least mentioned in the marvelous study, they couldn't show any difference. I would like to ask your opinion of the following: Do you think this striking difference in results is due to the design of the trial or you think that there is really a difference in one of the beta blockers?

<u>Dr. Sleight:</u>   I would say first of all, I think that the effect in

myocardial infarction is probably a class effect and I don't think there is any difference between the two beta blockers, but the word difference is in the trial. Their's was a much more complex and rigorous trial in a way and it took longer to get people in and there was a 4 hour difference if you notice in the mean time of onset, 5 hours versus 8.9 hours. That might have had a difference.

Dr. Ruberio: He also showed that there was no difference in beneficial effect if you separate the patients before and after 4 hours.

Dr. Sleight: Yes, I know, but perhaps I should have made it clearer that although we separated before and after 4 hours, which was one of the things that we had said in our protocol, we are going to do, in actual fact, most of the patients were in by 6 hours and so that wasn't a particularly discriminate dividing line.

Dr. Morganroth: Two years ago, I asked Dr. Temple this same question and in light of Dr. Hayes' remarks last night concerning resources and expenses for doing very large trials, when once we have a result of a trial, that a particular beta blocker has a well demonstrated claim, e.g. a decrease in the mortality in acute AMI patients what should the policy be concerning the study of other beta blockers? Or are we still at the point when each additional drug would have to be so tested in large trials.

Dr. Temple: Unfortunately, we haven't agreed that anything is effective early so we haven't had to leap off that precipice. There is a difference between what one's gut sensation is and what one thinks is likely to be true and what regulatory policy ought to be. You can be 95% sure that beta blockers will behave similarly. It is not clear to me that that entitles one to give an indication to a beta blocker as a class effect unless there really is quite a bit of data for several at least that show that these effects are in fact similar and even then, you could get into major arguments about how far to extend it. I mean for example, I think everyone would agree that if a drug had significant intrinsic sympathomimetic activity, that would be a whole new ball game. We don't know whether penetrance of the central nervous system matters. The evidence sort of is that it doesn't, since some drugs that do and some drugs that don't seem to have done all right. I don't think

we know completely whether the fact that the drug seemed to behave similarly
so far anyway in relatively late interventions, implies that they will behave
similarly in early interventions, although in all these cases, one is
inclined to think they will. My bias still is that in matters of life and
death of this kind, the drugs ought to be studied and that my own biases
and presumptions should be suppressed. I am not even sure that Dr. Sleight
and I would disagree on that.

Dr. Sleight: I don't think that we would disagree. If you were to take
beta blockers and their class effects, I think first of all you perhaps might
if I were a licensing authority, I would say that some things appear to be a
class effect. We will let through the ones that have actually done the work
and done the trial and the other ones will have to produce enough data to
satisfy me to at least look as though they are not harmful. I think you
might perhaps lower your thresholds a bit. I absolutely agree with you
though about ISA for example, because Richard Peter has proved all the trials
now that the European Australian Pindolol trial is out, it really does look
like that post-infarction ISA might not be quite such a good thing. It looks
like about a 10% benefit if you pool all the ISA blockers and about a 30%
benefit if you pool the non-ISA beta blockers after infarction so I would
agree with some caution there.

Dr. Turi: Let me just add one thing. We clearly already have lowered our
threshold. Nobody would insist once the point is established for one beta
blocker, I don't think anyone would insist on a placebo control trial, so
once you are into a positive control comparison, that represents a very
much lower standard of evidence and it really does mostly show that there
is nothing harmful going on. It is not a very strong standard of proof by
a long shot.

Dr. Temple: I think one might even question the relative ethics of the
placebo control trial in some of these settings. One point I would make in
terms of extrapolating to other beta blockers is that if one took the
timolol trial, and the metoprolol trial and automatically extended it for
example to propranolol without taking into account the history of trials with
that substance, which has been the most extensive, one might get perhaps the
wrong impression about the appropriate dosages. Before BHAT which gave

180-240 mg/day, there have been a number of relatively negative propranolol trials including one at 160 mg/day. I think that is absolute truth, there were differences in trial designs, certainly, it is clear that it is worth doing these trials if for no other reason than to be certain that the dosage forms are proper and that the administration, the time of administration and so on is correct.

Dr. Ruberio: Dr. Dern I was very glad to hear you emphasizing the issue that usually we miss people involved with infarct size reduction. When we have a myocardial infarction we really have two phenomena going on at the same time. One is the necrosis and the other is the fibrosis and as you well emphasized, sometimes we can influence one beneficially and the other one deleteriously. The analogy I make is with beta 1+ beta 2 receptors. You can block one without blocking the other or we can have a drug to block both but it is also dose dependent. You mentioned that there was some unpublished data where one dose didn't interfere with the healing process and my question is, in that one dose, did it not interfere with the healing process if they still could accomplish a reduction in the infarct size?

Dr. Dern: The studies you are referring to are studies in the dog, in which one dose was given intravenously and then at 6 hours an intramuscular dose was given. I think you have got difficulties with that and I have heard unofficially that similar studies with only the intravenous dose did not lead to such difficulties. I don't know how strongly to emphasize that, but in the current trials that we are now evaluating, the way the problem has been approached is to select an early small dose and get away from this business of repeated administration with the corticoids and then you get involved with the issue of time from onset of ischemia by stratification on that variable. The whole theme that runs through the glucocorticoid experimental and human experience up until the most recent trials is that these two variables, time from infarction and dosage frequency seem to be the most important and we will just have to see what the resultant of the trials is to take those things into account.

Dr. Loeb: I don't think there is serious question that amrinone has inotropic activity but I do take exception with the concept that in the intact patient by systemic hemodynamic measurements, one can make that assessment. Even at the small dosages of the preciseness of measurements, the effects of autonomic nervous system and compensatory adjustments as well as the possibility of release of stored catechols by any agent, I think makes it very difficult to make any assessment of direct inotropic effect. A way around that is to give a drug in very small doses intracoronary and then make measurements that directly relate to myocardial inotropic activity. In our dog lab with amrinone this method suggests that it is a direct inotropic or at least it has an inotropic effect independent of any systemic effects and it is also quite possible to do these kinds of measurements in the intact patient both without and with heart failure in the course of routine diagnostic catheterization. I think such studies really need to be done to clarify some of these issues. I would like to ask Dr. Temple to postulate whether or not the FDA would, and how they would approach, and what result would occur if digitalis were a new drug and being suggested as one for evaluation and approval.

Dr. Lipicky: Before you answer that, I wonder if you would educate me. If indeed one can conclude that a drug is an inotrope in isolated papillary muscle and in the dog lab, and clearly has no question that it changes the contractile force of the myocardium, what reason do you have to suspect that it would not in man?

Dr. Loeb: I don't have any reason that it isn't, but I think that issue has been raised and particularly in heart failure, the degree to which the diseased end stage failing heart can respond to an inotrope I think this is an issue that has been raised and one that could be dealt with in the framework of direct intracoronary administration in the intact human with heart failure during the course of other diagnostic procedures. There is nothing unique about that approach and I think it is one that would be a more direct way of getting that information.

Dr. Lipicky: Sure, but just to pursue the point for the moment. If there is no reason to suppose that something that you know is a positive inotrope should not be in man, that is if the myocardium has contractile proteins in the sarcosplasmic reticulum, it has something like a reasonable excitation contraction coupling mechanism, that in fact it ought to behave pretty much similarly to a chemical if there is a cell there. Why then although clearly one has to wonder about the what the relative contributions of a peripheral effect and the inotropic effect might be, would one want to question that the inotropic effect plays a role, or to what extent would that information be useful?

Dr. Loeb: It is difficult to speculate as to how basic mechanistic answers might be used down the road in clinical application. I think that if one is able to gain direct information about mechanisms of action that is accurate and is easily obtainable or relatively easily obtainable, that traditionally that information is worth obtaining. One doesn't always know how basic information will be applied in the future. Perhaps one need do nothing more than give a drug to a patient or group of patients and then count the patients that return to clinic three years later and count the ones that are buried. That might be the only real end result, but I think that we probably are doing a bit more than that, although perhaps we are doing a bit too much in some of these controlled studies in which the cost of the study escalates and the number of patients that enter this study decline as the complexity of the study increases, so that I think sometimes the end points may be more simple than some of the major endpoints. I can't really answer your question, but I think it is nice and important to have some concept from a physiologic point of view of how a drug works if one is contemplating using that drug in patients.

Dr. Lipicky: I don't disagree with your point but you are aware that the dp/dt with amrinone in heart failure patients has been measured and that there has been direct intracoranary administration of amrinone.

Dr. Loeb: Right, but as we see the new class of amrinone derivatives coming up, I think these questions may be raised. I am not advocating that tremendous amounts of money be spent in doing these studies, I am just suggesting that this is an approach which is probably a more direct and more accurate one than trying to assess it from systemic hemodynamics. We for instance studied and compared dobutamine to intravenous nitroprusside in all of the systemic effects. If you put the results side by side, there would be no way of knowing whether the effect was dobutamine or a nipride administration. It is very difficult.

<u>Dr. Temple</u>:   It seems to me that is the most important insight because as
Dr. Lipicky said initially, it feels like it might be bad to give an inotrope
to a person who has just had an acute myocardial infarction and it feels like
it might be better to give him a vasodilator. Well at least if what you give
him is an arterial vasodilator, it probably doesn't matter which one you give
him because they both end up with a very similar mechanism and if you measure
systolic intervals or if you measure anything you can measure hemodynamically
whether it is through internal compensations or what, they seem to do about
the same thing. That seems to be quite important.

<u>Dr. Loeb</u>:   The whole idea of the inotrope in acute myocardial
infarction is interesting. The catechols and the amrinone type drugs , I
think everybody accepts catechols as inotropes and also amrinone type drugs
as inotropes. They are different that digitalis and the digitalis
glycosides. None of the inotropes other than digitalis that I know of,
tends to slow the heart rate significantly when given to patients who have
heart failure and tachycardia. They may slow it slightly, but not to the
extent digitalis does, and yet digitalis is almost in many places reached a
point where many house staff officers are forbidden to use it in acute
myocardial infarction and other places it is used quite frequently. It is
probably the oldest drug about which we know the least and one perhaps
which I would be curious to know if it were a new drug, whether it would
have a chance of FDA approval.

<u>Dr. Sleight</u>: I have just read a very nice thesis by a chap called Bexton
from London who looked at about 20 human transplant patients and he used this
nice physiological preparation to distinguish between the direct effects of
drugs and the indirect effects as Bob Temple is suggesting. If you use a
vasodilator and as a result of that you get a reflex catecholamine release,
then it is not so much different from giving a drug which is a vasodilator
and an inotrope. He showed with this that nifedipine has two effects, that
it has a direct depressant effect upon the donor node and a reflex
sympathetic effect upon the recipient node, and I think it becomes very
difficult to separate these things and I would absolutely agree with what you
were saying in the need to be more precise in measurement to distinguish
between a positive inotropic effect and a reflex effect. You can't always
have transplant patients to do it on though.

Dr. Morganroth: Dr. Temple, once a drug has been on the market for decades, can the FDA remove that drug from having an approval status?

Dr. Temple: Sure, the question I assumed was not whether I thought there was sufficient information to put it on in the first place, but whether someone could do it properly. Let me answer both. Believe it or not we had to consider that question recently for various sort of boring beaurocratic reasons because we approved the new dosage form, not quickly but eventually of digitalis, so we had to prepare a summary basis of approval and we scanned the literature to try to extract from it two things that could credibly be called well controlled studies of the effects of digitalis for its various indications. We eventually did it, but the studies are anything but perfect in their design. There isn't anybody who has taken virgin patients with congestive heart failure and randomly assigned them to digitalis and nothing or diuretics plus digitalis and nothing or something that anybody would do if he were setting out to design the study. My guess is that if someone did such a study, it would turn out that digitalis can be shown to either increase exercise tolerance of N.Y. heart association classification or something of that kind. There was one reasonably persuasive study out of California in which people with a clear history of heart failure event (that is I believe they all have had to have pulmonary edema documented at some point and had been maintained on digitalis for a while were removed from it), and about half of them went into overt failure, and all of them had hemodynamic decompensation. Again, it is not exactly a perfect study, but it was really quite convincing. That convinces me at least reasonably well that there is at least some population of patients who if you choose them properly would be shown in a well controlled study to benefit from digitalis by a variety of generally accepted measures, so I think it would probably work out O.K. What also is clear from large quantitities of data that have been collected from people who were found to be on digitalis, is that the use of digitalis is sort of crazy, especially in England I gather, where most of these studies have come from, because perhaps as many as 90% of the patients are on for some peculiar reason such as a predominant kidney problem, or they were put on it for a course of pneumonia and the old dogma, once on digitalis always on digitalis has led to maintenance of digoxin in people who plainly didn't need it. When studies are done where peole are withdrawn from digitalis and there is no attempt to find people who really should have been on it, you conclude that it hasn't done any good for most of the people who were on it which I am sure is true also. I think it would probably make it through the conventional process.

Dr. Sleight: I would like to reply not quite as fiercely as the noise is off. I defend England. The use of digitalis is not very high in England. If you took acute myocardial infarction, one of the interesting things about our ISIS trial is that we have asked the patient, the simple form on discharge says what drugs are they on at discharge, and we have a 10% sample at 6 months follow-up of all the population to see what drugs they are on at 6 months. The interesting thing is that some countries know things that other countries don't. Like in Scandinavia, I think 47% of the population are on digoxin after discharge from acute myocardial infarction. In England it is 4%. In Italy 50% also are on anti-platelet agents and also in Italy, an enormous number, something like 50% get intravenous nitrates during the coronary care and it is just staggeringly different from country to country and I think we have a real education problem.

Dr. Lee: Dr. Sleight, you mentioned a certain percentage of your Atenolol patients in whom you got into some sort of difficulty early on with Atenolol. Did you talk about the percentage of patients in whom you got into some difficulties what the difficulties were, and what was the outcome of that episode. Did you have to use agonists?

Dr. Sleight: Yes, protocol deviations occurred in I think something like 33 or so of both groups in that the patients who were randomized and analyzed in the non-beta blocked group, 33 of them got beta blockers during the course of their hospital stay, because the clinicians who were looking after them thought they needed them and about 33 or 37 of the beta blocker group did not complete the course of treatment and that was usually in the vast majority of them. They were sufficiently hypotensive and bradycardic that it worried the physician and they did not continue with the oral treatment. But I think the use of inotropes was about 4 or 5 in the beta blocker group only and so for the vast majority of them, all they did was either stop the treatment or in about I think 15 cases, they used atropine. It was not a problem except in 1 or 2 patients where they had to use more aggressive inotropic therapy

and actually in those patients, they fortunately came out alive, perfectly
well with as it turned out rather small infarcts. It has not been a real
problem and I can say that now with some confidence because of this very much
larger study where they particularly look for that. I would emphasize that
these are selected patients who look like good risk patients. They are not
by any means the largest proportion of people who come into the coronary care
unit. They would be about 25 to 30% of our coronary care unit intake. So
they are good risk patients. They are not clammy looking patients.

Dr. Turi: We also took good risk patients like Dr. Sleight and we gave them
beta blockade somewhat later so that they aren't quite the same. We were
very prudent with propranolol. We gave 0.1 mg/kg, but we gave it in 3
divided doses and stopped if the heart rate fell below 45. They really had
very little if any problem. I think 1 patient developed heart failure and
there was a very low incidence of bradyarrhythmias.

Dr. Bush: I have a comment relating the the previous discussion and
that is I think it is worth noting that a few years back in acute MI's in
animal experiments that while ouabain did not exacerbate any effects of
ischemic injury in that setting, isoproterenol did so I think it is important
what kind of inotropic stimulation one uses. More recently one of my
colleagues showed using a different index of ischemic injury,
(intramyocardial CO_2 tension) that again ouabain did not increase the
extent of ischemic injury, but an increase in heart rate did and that
increase in heart rate was induced by pacing. Based on those comments, I
would be interested in asking any of the panelists, to what extent data from
these types of experiments are heeded or acknowledged and or acknowledged?

Dr. Temple: I think what you said is obviously correct. I think anybody
would worry about an intervention that deliberately increased heart rate a
lot. We spent a lot of time arguing about atropine on a basis just like that
and the people who opposed a widespread use of atropine anyway were worried
about exactly that thing that with an increase in heart rate seems to be
about the worse thing you can do at the time of an infarction. But of course
it is not clear what that has to do with. Isoproterenol increased the heart
rate for a bunch of reasons, the main one of which is probably not the fact
that it is a vasodilator, so that it remains probably true that choosing

between an arterial dilator and an inotropic agent, that may still be
substantially indistinguishable in their hemodynamic effects. I think people
who design trials do think about things like that.

Dr. Sleight: Most doctors take very little notice of experiments and
clinical trials I am sad to tell.

Dr. Capone: I would like to address a question to Dr. Sleight,
specifically with regard to the methodology of randomization. Since your
study was non-blinded is it possible that some of the differences between
your trial with atenolol and the MILIS study is related to the non-blinded
nature? I am interested in whether this is possible? I am interested in
whether the control group was approached in the same way in terms of getting
informed consent and whether diffferences in approach might in some way have
affected the outcome.

Dr. Sleight: They were both obviously approached in the same way and told
there was a flip of the coin as to whether they got this new treatment or the
routine treatment was the way we approached that. I don't think there is any
difference in their approach to the patients. We didn't select a control
group who refused to come into the study. The question of blinding I think
is an important question and one can't absolutely answer it, except to say
that the end point that we measured, the CK-MB, they were all done in batches
blinded in another laboratory, away from our hospital in large numbers at a
time, and I don't think without knowledge of which group they were in. The
same was done about the analysis of the ECG score. I think that is all I can
say about it except that the next question is could it have influenced the
drugs that they got subsequently? The amount of vrosemide given is possible.
The only thing I can say is that the trialists were not actually looking
after the vast majority of the patients because all of the attending
physicians in different sort of firms were looking after their own patients
in this trial and if I had been another physician, I think I would have
tended to give more vrosemide to a patient who had had a beta blocker rather
than the last. I think that would have been any bias might have actually
gone the other way in that particular case. For the other drugs, the use of
digoxin and so on was so little that I don't think it really had any material
effect. It was more used in the controls than in the atenolol group, but I

wouldn't make a great deal of that. It is always a problem about whether you
double blind a thing or whether you are just double blinding yourself. It is
a placebo effect again on the trialist because I do believe, there it is very
obvious when you give an intravenous beta blocker to people. I am interested
to hear what Dr. Turi has to say about that. Maybe they looked at it and saw
if they could guess they had given propranolol or not.

Dr. Turi: I think it is misleading to assume that people did not know they
were given propranolol. The hyuluronidase portion is clearly blinded. Same
problem with the glucose-insulin-potassium studies. It is really basically
impossible to hide the method or approach. I think one potential thing to
emphasize about the MILIS study is that the kind of rigorous control with the
use of other medications is nevertheless important, particularly the
avoidance of all nitrates. I think there are a variety of issues why it is
impossible to compare these two studies.

Dr. Morganroth: Let's assume that the ISIS study comes out showing that
intravenous atenolol has a clear cut effect on mortality and let's assume
that there is an ultra-short acting beta blocker that might be available and
might be worth studying because of the issues Dr. Sleight raised and that the
adverse reactions could be markedly improved. I am still confused as to how
I would set up such a trial, because I do agree with what Dr. Temple said
that a class action claim for beta blockers even particularly in the acute
setting is premature. Therefore, if I had an ultra short-acting beta blocker
and I wanted to get it approved for the use in acute myocardial infarction
patients, would we need a study that showed it had some positive benefit or
effect. In this country I suspect we couldn't do a placebo controlled study
on this use. How do we deal with this problem?

Dr. Sleight: I think it would be impossible to do a positive trial between
a short-acting and a long-acting beta blocker. Supposing the ISIS study
comes up positive and then you have a short-acting one adn you say this might
be nicer because in the very small number of people with an adverse effect,
it will stop quicker. I think in practical terms, that is probably not too
important, but supposing we think it is important, then I think you would
have to do a trial, and if I were the FDA I would say that you have to have
say 1000 patients against it and you have to showthat is no worse. I think

you just have to test the null hypothesis.

Dr. Morganroth: So essentially you are looking at safety, not efficacy.

Dr. Sleight   Yes, I would be looking at safety I think.

Dr. Temple: I would agree. You would learn. There are two parts. I don't think one would insist that you show that there is a gain from the short acting one, but you would want to be sure with the regimen with the short-acting one as the introduction to the longer acting drug was of comparable effectiveness, or at least not overtly worse. I think that would require a fairly good sized positive control trial but not so big that you would be able to show an actual favorable difference. The kind of effectiveness data you get from a trial that fails to show a difference and is of a limited kind. The reason I think you would probably need a fairly large trial. I guess it is hard to assert that a trial substantially smaller than the placebo control trial would be very persuasive. It is a sticky issue.

Dr. Sleight: I would say that if we show this is an effect, then I am a manufacturer, so I can say this without any shadow of doubt, I would be very happy if somebody else did a 1000 patients and showed that it wasn't dangerous. I wouldn't want them to do 10,000 patients again. I think it would be ridicuous.

Dr. Temple: The question is why should one move from a study that clearly showed a beneficial effect on mortality assuming that it indeed came out that way. Shouldn't one need quite a good reason for saying that an alternative regimen is just as good. I mean it seems to me that the down side is very large, and the gain to anybody is very small, unless there is for example in that population, quite a large number of people who get into trouble from that first dose. If there is as you said in the first case, not much trouble from the first dose, and if there is trouble you can handle it anyway, there isn't any tremendous incentive to get a short-acting one even though as Dr. Morganroth says, it makes some sense. I would think you would want a fairly convincing reason to put another regimen out there especially when there would be this implication that it had an advantage which wouldn't be true, wouldn't be known and take people off the regimen that have been studied. I think that is a very big step when you are taking about mortality.

Dr. Lessem: I have two small questions to Dr. Turi. In your study of nifedipine, I would like to know whether you had any concomitant medication that could have changed the results of your study? The second question is would you have preferred a large trial with verapamil now that verapamil has some different actions than nifedipine has?

Dr. Turi: First as far as concomitant medication, we made major efforts to avoid concomitant medication keeping in mind that other vasodilators might muddle these considerably. So that patients who were on nitrates were withdrawn from nitrates unless we felt that the dose of nitrates was such that it might be harmful to acutely discontinue it, but keeping in mind I think the conclusions of most of this panel, that there are precious few drugs which are clearly efficacious in acute myocardial infarction. We felt that by and large, it was prudent and reasonable to not have patients on other medications. Patients on beta blockade were maintained but the dose was not increased, assuming that they were on substantial doses. So I do not believe, we were very prudent about the use of other medications and there were very few variations in that. As far as trials of verapamil, verapamil has a theoretical additional benefit of changing the VF threshold and it theoretically might also be very efficacious calcium blocker in acute infarction. The studies that were done with verapamil have not been overwhelmingly positive. Those are the two answers to your question. There is also a point to came to mind. The absence of any mortality at all in our control group is somewhat bizarre when you consider that there were 100 control patients and had no mortality in the first two weeks, makes some of that mortality data somewhat suspect. We did look at the 62 patients who were considered eligible and were not randomized because they refused or their physicians refused and one could consider those also to be a fairly good parallel to the placebo group, although if your physician or yourself are a type A personality or whatever the reason people refuse protocols, maybe that is not the perfect comparison, but there was about a 5% mortality rate in that group so it is a little difficult to assess mortality in that sense. In answer to your question I had great hopes for verapamil and have been disappointed with what I have seen in terms of studies done so far. Dr. Sleight do you want to comment?

Dr. Sleight: No, except to agree with you that just to enter a trial is to confer immortality to the patient which is one of the difficulties for all trialists. The Danish trial is over 1000 patients showed a slightly adverse effect of Verapamil. There was not a hint of any benefit for it. I think that is correct. It is not published yet that I know.

Dr. Goldstein: Two things I would like to add. One is relative to blinding. We looked at blinding in BHAT and we fortunately had an opportunity to use the same instrument at close-out that we used in the aspirin- myocardial infarction study. In the aspirin myocardial infarction study, there was a very even split in terms of patients having any idea about their drug therapy. There was really no bias whatsoever. It was amazingly right down the middle, but with BHAT there was clearly a turn towards people perceiving they were on a beta blocker. Although it wasn't all the way, I believe that 60-75% of people thought they were on the drug and there was some recognition clearly that people who took the drug were more aware or perceived being on a drug than the placebo group. We also looked at the question of digitalis in BHAT. The question is you know there have been a couple of studies looking at digitalis in post-infarction patients. Probably the largest one is the group carried out in the multicenter trial headed by Art Moss and that group showed that in people with premature beats, the mortality rate was considerably higher in those people on digitalis as compared to those without it. We looked at digitalis in BHAT and I think there are about 10% of people who were on digitalis in the trial. Some for no reason at all as alluded to and some because they actually had congestive heart failure. It is obviously difficult to separate out the mortality effects of digitalis in people with congestive heart failure, but clearly the people who were on digitalis and congestive heart failure had a higher mortality rate and the digitalis seemed to add to that mortality rate. In those people who were on digitalis without congestive heart failure, again the mortality rate was higher on digitalis, but it didn't really reach levels of statistical significance but it was clearly a trend in that direction. It does raise some suspicions as to how safe it is to give digitalis in post-infarction patients.

Dr. Turi: A question for you Dr. Goldstein. Do you think that some of the digitalis trials, Dr. Moss' among others have been BHAT studies in reverse? That has not been a fact that has been analyzed in any of those assessments of defect of digitalis and the curves look like upside down BHAT curves. In other words, these patients, the ones that went home on digitalis might have been excluded or might have been patients who would not have been on propranolol. I guess what I am asking you is is it possible that the patients on digitalis, not being on propranolol means that they are really suffering the effects of lack of beta blockade?

Dr. Goldstein: Interesting. I have to think that one through.

Dr. Loeb: Dr. Sleight, I think you alluded to something like 35 or 40% of patients in the average CCU would get in to the beta blocker study and these are the good risk patients. By good risk I assume that these are patients least likely to die either during the acute phase, probably during the first year after their infarct which leaves 2/3 of the highest risk patients for which we really don't have guidelines in terms of prophylactic or continuous beta blocker therapy, primarily because one feels that the beta blockers might be dangerous. In these less than ideal patients then, a short acting beta blocker might be a useful means of increasing or at least testing the safety of administration of beta blockers which then could have the result of increasing that population of patients who it might be very safe or even desirable to put them on long term beta blockers but who are currently not probably not receiving beta blocker therapy, so I would like to know how you feel about that.

Dr. Sleight: There are two different sort of questions it seems to me. If you talk about long-term beta blockade, there is no doubt that the Hanstein high risk beta blocker study post-infarction beginning I think at 4 days post-infarction, showed without a shadow of a doubt that even if you had heart failure, that you were better to go onto a beta blocker and have your heart failure treated at the same time and have the protection of the beta blocker. That seemed without doubt. I wouldn't have any hesitation about witholding beta blockade for people with mild to moderate heart failure. I would actually actively put them on it. But a day or two before they are discharged. I think there is a window in between the first few hours and 2 or 3 days. I have no proof of this, but I have a sort of gut feeling, that there is a window in intravenous blockade or oral beta blockade would be bad news. I think if you can get in early, our evidence so far suggests that you do reduce infarct size and you don't commit mayhem and there are some beneficial effects, but in the middle I would be more cautious. Now it may be that we are being ultra cautious at the very beginning and that if we could get in early at sick people, then maybe IV beta blockade would be O.K. but I would be jolly hesitant about it.

Dr. Turi: It does raise the question of whether rather than saying therapy should be begun with this new very short acting drug, you could think of it as a way to test for beta blocker tolerance. That is obviously a somewhat easier study to do.

Dr. Sleight: But you might not have long enough to test for it is my point.

Karen Heller: I have a question that is similar to this. If you were hypothetically to receive data that you believe that showed that a regular preparation of propranolol had an effect on either short term mortality or long term mortality, what would you like to see in terms of approving a long acting formulation or a slow release formulation of propranolol? Do you want that data repeated or just show equivalent area under the curve data?

Dr. Temple: We had a similar problem regarding the BHAT trial. As everybody knows the BHAT trial was done with a 3 times a day regimen and there is not a whole lot of point of ducking your head into the sand and approving a 3 times a day regimen and not saying anything about another regimen because you know a) people won't use it or b) they will give a BID regimen anyway. So we spent a lot of time with propranolol kinetic curves and looking at just what the difference was in the blood levels that occurred when you gave a similar dose BID and TID and eventually sucked in our guts and at least commented favorably on the possibility of in the labeling a twice daily regimen. There is an elaborate, perhaps slightly defensive rationale for why that is an O.K. thing to do, that we think makes good sense. To then go further and try to do the same thing with the long acting regimen which is just very different. It does plainly work in hypertension and works in angina, but it is a very different kinetic profile from what you get when you give it either 3 times a day or twice a day. My own reaction would be that is pulling a little bit too far from the data base that you have and for reasons that I gave earlier, I would be very uncomfortable doing that. Obviously, many physicians will reach their own conclusions about such things and I have no doubt that atenolol, nadolol, etc. are being used for prevention of post-infarction mortality whether there is a clear data base or not.

Dr. Lipicky: I might elaborate on this point that I thought I was trying to make with respect to amrinone but it apparently was missed. That is when we were thinking about long acting beta blocker, we came to the conclusion, that because its absorption characteristics were different and because it had first pass metabolism that there was no way that one could relate the dose that one needed to administer to the experience that one knew about with the immediate release dosage form and came to the conclusion that the sustained release dosage form needed to have some kind of empirical dose range in study that simply put it in the ball park of what it is that one had some feeling for and I emphasize the fact that it is a feeling for the immediate release dosage form because in fact I have a great deal of difficulty finding any reasonable dose-response relationships even for the immediate release dosage forms. Then when one comes to an efficacy trial that indeed shows some change in mortality and can't ascribe the mortality effect to any known effect of the drug, that is, is it this,this or this, let alone to how whatever the effect of the drug is that the mortality is due to, how that effect is related to dose and then comes and says, now I want to change the way in which I am going to administer the drug and hope that there is a chance in being able to through some contortion of reasoning get away with that, I just don't see how that is possible.

Dr. Sleight: I am staggered. I mean I really would take the opposite view point. I think that if you have got a slow release formulation that is shown to be effective in hypertension and angina and then you say there is something magically different about this 3 times a day beta blockers, I can't see it.

Dr. Temple: What about a trial of propranolol at 40 mg 4 times a day that failed to show effect. Are you certain that is not a result of the dose. How does one know that.

Dr. Sleight: I think you would want to have an effective dose, but to say to give it 3 times a day and then put the thing in the slow release and have the same blood levels shown.

Dr. Temple: You don't get the same blood levels.

Dr. Sleight: You have got them down more you mean?

Dr. Temple: They are very different. They are substantially lower toward the evening hours. There is enough residual left to still be effective in certain measurements, but I think that is the point we are making. They are very different from the blood levels that are achieved.

Dr. Lipicky: Tell me what it is that you would try to match. The area under the curve, the trough level, the peak level, the root mean square? What is it that this sustained release formulation should match if what you are trying to do is come up with the appropriate immediate release?

Dr. Sleight: If you wanted a crude thing, I would rather go on heart rate than anything else.

Dr. Temple: My reaction would be that if the long-acting really did sort of split the difference of the rises and falls of the three times a day regimen, probably we wouldn't have so much problem with it. It doesn't do that or come particularly close to it. It is similar for the first 12-16 hours and then it is considerably lower.

Dr. Sleight: You are meaning to say that it is probably better to have some peaks and troughs.

Dr. Temple: No you might make a good case for giving the slow release for the first 12 hours or something like that but I mean a once a day regimen with the slow release gives you blood levels and isoproterenol responses and anything else you care to measure that are very different from giving half the dose at night. They are not the same. If they were really the same or were sort of in the middle, I don't think we would have any trouble, but that is not what they look like.

Dr. Sleight: I think you are getting a bit nit-picking Bob.

21

TRANSLUMINAL CORONARY ANGIOPLASTY

S. GOLDBERG

After extensive experience with transluminal dilatation
of peripheral arterial stenoses, Gruentzig in 1977 performed
successful percutaneous balloon coronary angioplasty in man[1]
Since his original report, the technique of transluminal
balloon dilatation of coronary arterial stenoses has become
a widespread and effective technique for the relief of myocardial ischemia due to severe fixed coronary atheroscle-
rosis[2,3]. Preliminary experience with balloon angioplasty
was collected by the National Heart, Lung, and Blood Institute
voluntary registry and the initial encouraging results
reported in patients with predominantly single vessel disease
have led investigators to extend the procedure to higher risk
subgroups of patients. In this section the indications,
techniques,and results of coronary angioplasty will be
reviewed.

Indications for Coronary Angioplasty

Patients initially described as being suitable for
angioplasty were those with objective evidence for myocardial
ischemia who had failed a medical regimen, and were
candidates for bypass surgery. On coronary angiography, the ideal stenosis was a critical proximal lesion
which was concentric and noncalcified.

Important improvements in catheter design along with
increased physician experience have permitted a careful
extension of guidelines to include patients with more unstable clinical conditions and complex anatomy. Currently
angioplasty is being performed on more distal, eccentric and

229

calcified coronary lesions. In addition the technique has been applied with reasonable success to patients with totally occluded coronary arteries[5], to those with multivessel disease[6], and to patients who have previously undergone bypass graft surgery. A further application of transluminal coronary angioplasty has been in patients with acute evolving myocardial infarction[7-9].

An important advance allowing for extension of the technique has been the development of a dilatation catheter system which has as a critical component independently moveable and exchangeable guide wires.

Technique

Initially, transluminal coronary angioplasty was carried out via fixed guide wire catheter systems (Fig. 1).

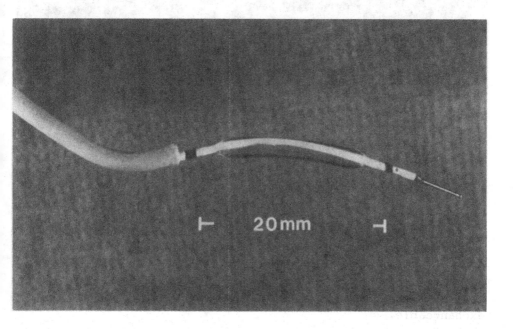

Figure 1. The early fixed guide wire balloon dilatation catheter in guiding catheter. From Greenspon and Goldberg - Cardiovascular Clinics.

These early catheters were double lumen 4 French devices.

One lumen was used for pressure monitoring through a distal
port as well as contrast injections, while the second lumen
connected to the balloon itself. A non-moveable, flexible,
straight or J tipped guide wire was fastened to the distal end
of the dilatation catheter.

A most important development has been the introduction of
an angioplasty system which consists of a dilatation catheter
through which a soft, steerable guide wire can be passed and
moved independently of the dilatation catheter (Fig. 2).

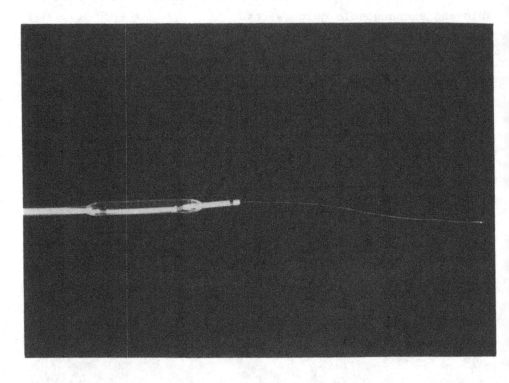

Figure 2. The newer moveable guide wire-dilatation catheter
system. The guide wire is independently moveable and
exchangeable.

The use of this system allows for safer passage through tight,
eccentric stenoses or even totally occluded coronary arteries[6]
In addition, pressure monitoring through the guiding catheter
(seated in the ostium of the coronary artery to be dilated),
and the distal port of the dilatation catheter permits

measurement of the gradient across the stenosis before and after balloon inflation.

Guiding catheters are available in a variety of shapes and are either 8 or 9 French (Fig. 3).

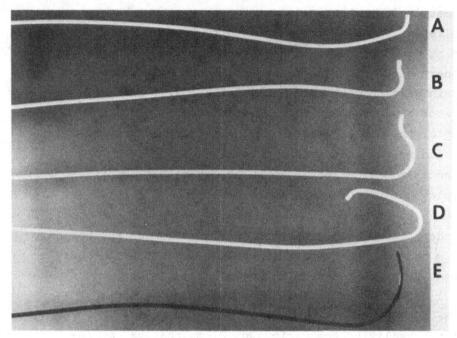

Figure 3. Variety of guiding catheters used in angioplasty.

Once the guiding catheter is seated in the coronary ostium, diagnostic angiograms are performed. The practice in our laboratory has been to inject intracoronary nitroglycerin, (approximately 200 ug) into the coronary to be dilated. This, in addition to pretreatment with nifedipine, (usually 20 mg sublingual), promotes coronary vasodilation and decreases the risk of coronary spasm during subselective coronary catheter manipulation. Adequate anticoagulation is critical, and heparin,(10,000 units) is administered prior to insertion of the dilating catheter. Frequent monitoring of the anti-coagulation status by means of the activated coagulation time using a hemochron[R] permits adjustment of the heparin dose. Proper seating of the guiding catheter relative to the coronary ostium is an important step in the angioplasty procedure. It is not satisfactory to achieve only an adequate dye injection

into the coronary artery, rather the operator must be satisfied
that the geometric orientation of the guiding catheter will
permit safe passage of the guide wire-dilatation system into
the ostium of the coronary artery and through the stenosis to
be dilated. Special care is taken to prevent "wedging" of the
guiding catheter in the coronary ostium with reduction of
coronary blood flow and subsequent myocardial ischemia.
Certain guiding catheter configurations will also help the
operator in subsequent passage of stenoses. For
example, the Amplatz configuration is particularly useful in
approaching left circumflex coronary lesions. In some
instances modification of approach may become important; for
example, the use of the brachial approach is helpful in
dilating right coronary artery and bypass graft stenoses.
Consideration of the geometric configuration of the coronary
ostium relative to the aorta, the portion of the coronary artery
segment proximal to the stenosis and the distal coronary anatomy
are all features taken into account before selection
of the appropriate components of the dilatation
system. Realizing the various problems that may be en-
countered during the dilatation procedure prior to undertaking
catheter selection is important in maximizing success rate.
Other noteworthy factors include careful scrutiny of the
region of the stenosis itself with reference to bends,
calcification, side branch vessels, degree of eccentricity,
and the severity of the stenosis itself.

After the operator is satisfied with the guiding
catheter position and the pressure tracings from the guiding
catheter, it is time to insert the dilating catheter-guide
wire system. A variety of dilating catheters are available
with different balloon sizes. The balloons vary in size
from 2.0 to 4.0 mm in inflated diameter and are usually 25 mm
in length. Metallic markers indicate the position of the
balloon segment during fluoroscopy. The "deflated profile"
of the balloon dilating catheters also differs depending on
the manufacturer. A variety of guide wires is available,

(Fig. 4) each with different characteristics and "trade-offs": The United States Catheter and Instrument (USCI) steerable wire, for example, is 0.016 inches in diameter, is highly radiopaque, and steerable.

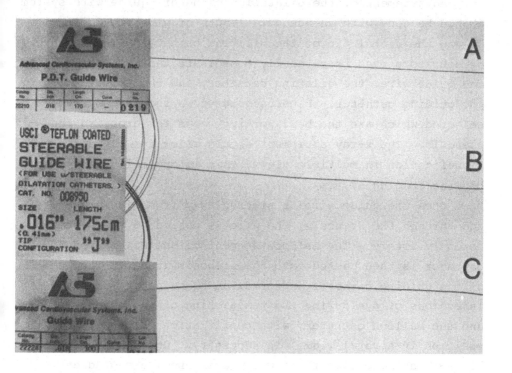

Figure 4. Types of moveable guide wires - each with different characteristics and "trade-offs".

It is somewhat stiffer than the Advanced Catheter System, (ACS) 0.018 inch "floppy" wire, which is much less radiopaque except for the distal tip; however, the floppiness of the ACS wire is especially useful in crossing tight, eccentric stenosis or finding a path through totally occluded coronary arteries. The latter also has very little chance of causing dissection; the "tradeoff" of using this "floppy" wire, of course, is that it is much less steerable. In addition, pressure measurements with this wire in place are not easily obtainable, and once a stenosis is crossed an exchange should be made for another wire (the pressure, dye, torque (PDT) of

ACS or steerable USCI) to obtain distal coronary pressure. A
300 cm "floppy" exchange wire is particularly useful in the
circumstance of having to use more than one dilating balloon
catheter to achieve a satisfactory dilatation.

Advancement of the dilatation catheter--guide wire system
should be done with an adequate length of wire protruding
beyond the distal tip of the dilating catheter. The operator
or operators need to carefully coordinate the movement of
the guide wire, the dilating catheter, and the position of
the guiding catheter. Fluoroscopic views should be pre-
selected which are the best working views for crossing the
stenosis. The x-ray equipment should allow for rapid
visualization in multiple views; this is optimally done with
biplane imaging systems.

Once the guide wire is steered away from side branches
and through the stenosis, the wire is passed to the distal
coronary artery. The balloon segment of the dilatation
catheter is then passed into the stenosis itself. The use
of the guiding catheter and/or dilating catheter for test
injections of dye during the positioning of the guide wire
and the balloon catheter, with confirmation of proper
position in several views, is necessary. Once the guide
wire--dilating catheter are well positioned, the gradient
across the stenosis can be measured (with certain guide
wire-catheter combinations) (Fig. 5) and balloon inflation can
take place.

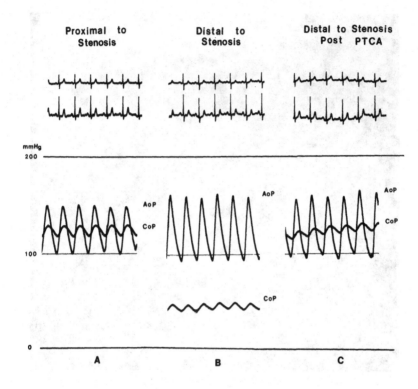

Figure 5. Example of transluminal pressure gradient measurement. In the left panel, simultaneous arterial pressure and
coronary pressure with dilating catheter proximal to stenosis.
In the middle panel - a transluminal gradient is recorded as
the catheter is passed through the stenosis. After the lesion
is dilated, the distal coronary pressure rises substantially
and the gradient is markedly reduced (right panel). From
Greenspon and Goldberg - Cardiovascular Clinics.

We prefer the use of a hand held inflation device, but the

mounted gun devices are acceptable as well. It is our

practice to begin with gradual inflation constantly watching

the shape of the balloon. We look specifically for the "dog

bone" effect (Fig. 6-9) present when the dilating balloon

engages the stenoses at lower inflation pressures.

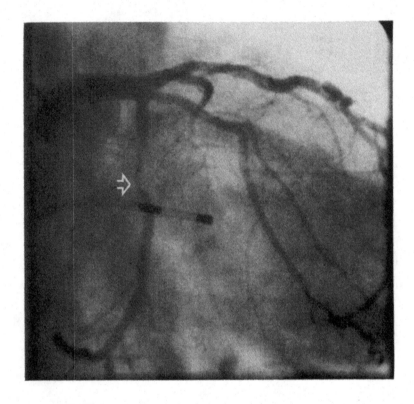

Figure 6 a) Left coronary angiogram showing a severe eccentric stenosis
in the left circumflex artery in a patient with severe rest angina.

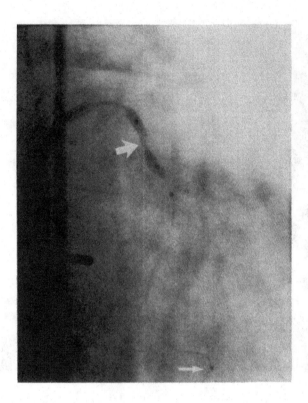

Figure 6 b) The dilatation catheter is well positioned within the stenosis and at the beginning of inflation. The "dog bone" effect is noted on the balloon (heavy arrow). This is caused by the stenosis restricting outward balloon expansion. The floppy wire is seen in the distal circumflex system (lighter arrow).

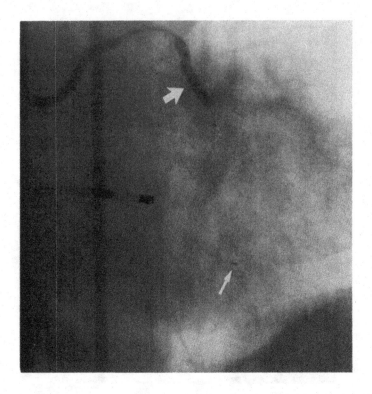

Figure 6 c) Appearance of the balloon at higher inflation pressures - note the disappearance of the "dog bone" effect, indicating that the stenosis has been dilated.

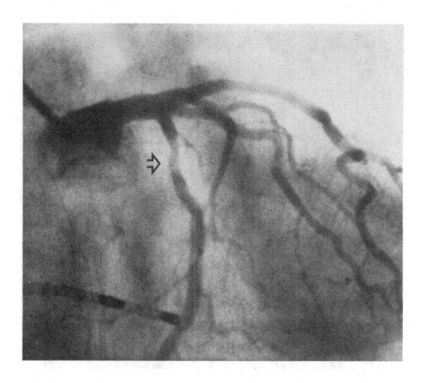

Figure 6 d) Result after dilatation. There is marked improvement in lumen diameter. Typical hazy appearance is noted (arrow).

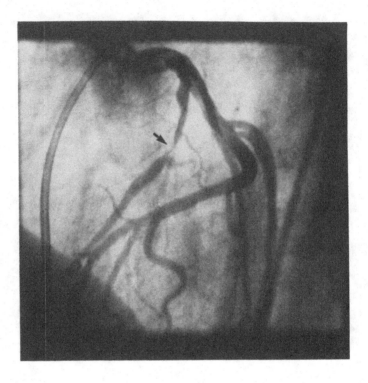

Figure 7 a) Left coronary angiogram of a 38 year old man with prior subendocardial infarction and post infarct angina· there is a 95% left anterior descending artery stenosis (arrow).

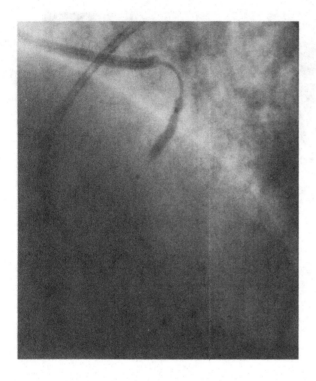

Figure 7 b) Inflation of balloon in stenosis.

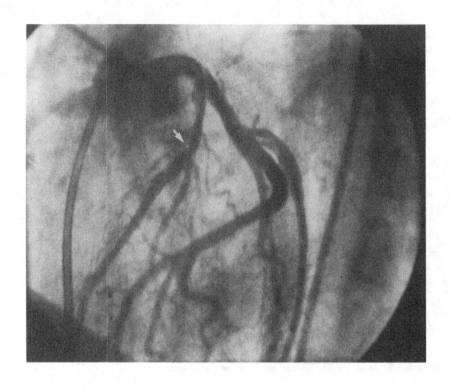

Figure 7 c) Result after angioplasty showing only residual luminal irregularity in the left anterior descending artery (arrow).

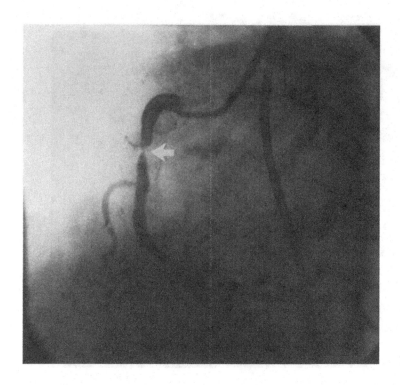

Figure 8 a) Severe right coronary segmental stenosis.

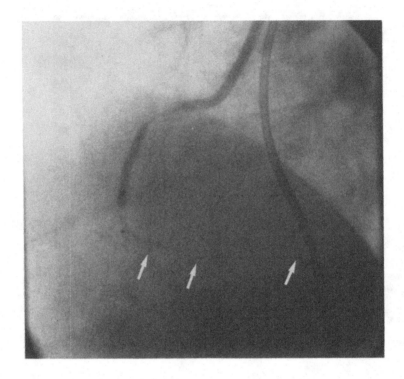

Figure 8 b) Balloon inflated in stenosis; note position of floppy wire in distal vessel (3 light arrows).

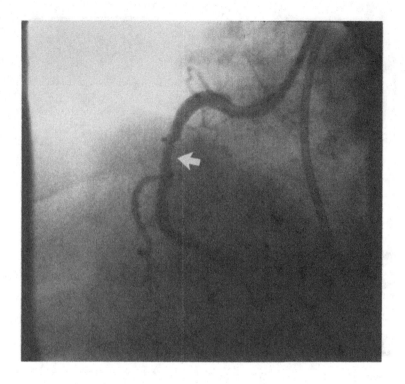

Figure 8 c) Result showing reduction of severe stenosis to luminal irregularity.

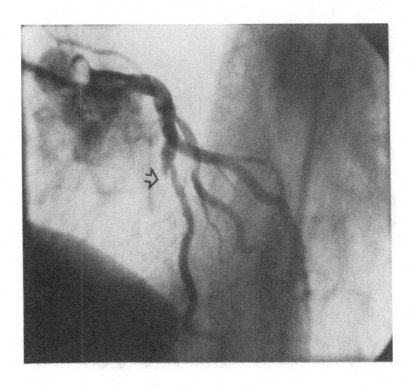

Figure 9 a) Left coronary angiogram of 52 year old man during acute
evolving anteroseptal myocardial infarction. There is total occlusion
of the left anterior descending coronary artery (arrow).

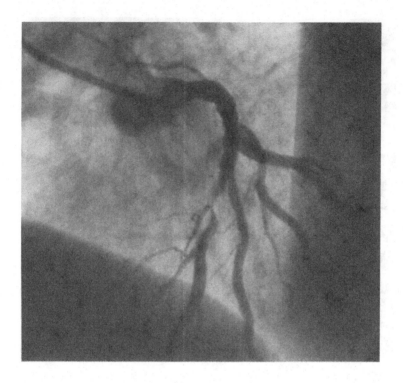

Figure 9 b) After the administration of intracoronary streptokinase, there is restoration of antegrade left anterior descending flow. A 95% stenosis remains at the site of prior thrombotic occlusion.

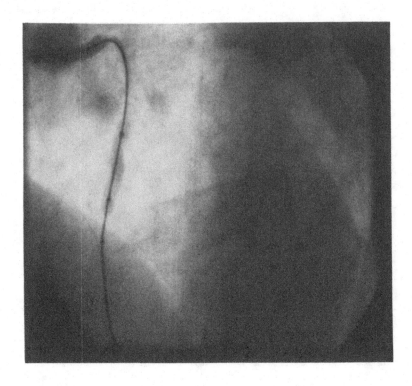

Figure 9 c) Several days following successful streptokinase therapy dilatation was performed.

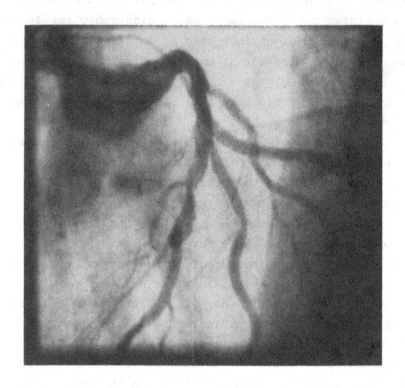

Figure 9 d) Final result showing marked improvement in lumen diameter.

Careful checking of the "dog bone" helps assure proper positioning of the balloon relative to the stenosis. With gradually increasing inflation pressure the "dog bone" disappears and the pressure at which this occurs is a guide to the softness or resistance of the lesion. Recently, we have performed longer inflations at higher pressures. Generally our first inflation is done for 30 seconds with constant arterial pressure and EKG monitoring, and we watch for the development of chest pain and/or ST segment elevation.

After the "dog bone" has disappeared, we deflate the balloon
and recheck the gradient and angiographic flow. Inflations
are repeated with gradually increasing inflation pressure
until a satisfactory hemodynamic and angiographic result
occurs. A final gradient less than 15 mm Hg is desirable.
We leave the guide wire across the stenosis and in the distal
vessel for approximately 30 minutes following the final balloon
inflation and during this time period, check for any change
in the magnitude of the gradient. A fall in distal coronary
pressure recorded through the tip of the dilatation catheter
in the 30 minutes following the last inflation may signal
coronary dissection. If this occurs, we repeat the dye
injection and, if appropriate, reinflate the balloon with a
long, low pressure inflation in an attempt to "tack down"
the dissection. Another cause for a drop in distal coronary
pressure may be the development of coronary spasm which can
be treated by intracoronary nitroglycerin injection. Balloon
inflation is repeated until there is no further gain in distal
coronary pressure, and the angiographic result appears
satisfactory. We attempt to increase the inflation time to
45-90 seconds or longer, if feasible, as preliminary evidence
suggests that long inflations may increase the primary success
rate and perhaps reduce the restenosis rate. If all appears
well after the 30 minute period, we remove the guide wire--
dilatation balloon catheter system and repeat the coronary
angiograms in multiple views. Typically, a certain amount
of "haziness" is present in the area of dilatation;
occasionally small dissections are clinically visible. In
certain instances, there maybe a suboptimal or ambigious
result. In this latter circumstance the hemodynamic measurements made across the coronary stenosis assume critical
clinical significance. Coronary dissection which causes
abrupt vessel closure usually does so in the first 30 minutes
after the last balloon inflation. Any patient who
develops an increasing stenosis gradient along with electrocardiographic and/or clinical evidence of myocardial ischemia

is immediately taken for bypass surgery.

Once dilatation is successfully accomplished, the patient is returned to the coronary care unit for 24 hours. We maintain patients on aspirin and persantine indefinitely and nifedipine and nitrates for six months. Stress electrocardiography is repeated in the two week period following successful angioplasty, and coronary angiography is repeated 6-12 months after angioplasty or sooner if indicated. Restenosis when it occurs, usually does so in the first 3-6 months.

Results and Directions of Angioplasty

In 1979 the National Heart Lung and Blood Institute (NHLBI) established a voluntary registry to assess the efficacy of transluminal coronary angioplasty. In the most recent report the results of 3,079 patients undergoing the procedure were analyzed[4]. Briefly, the findings may be summarized as follows. The patients were predominantly male (77%) with a mean age of 53.5 years. Twenty-six percent (26%) of patients were in Canadian Heart Class 4, 37% were in Class 3, 28% in Class 2, 4% in Class 1, and 5% had no symptoms. Seventy-three percent (73%) of patients had single vessel disease, 25% had multivessel disease, and 2% had left main coronary artery disease. The angiographic success rate was somewhat higher in males than females (68% vs. 63%), and the overall complication rate was 19% in males and 27% in females. In-hospital deaths occurred in 0.7% of men and 1.8% of women. The major complications included coronary dissection/occlusion/ spasm occurring in 10.4%, myocardial infarction occurring in 5.5%, ventricular tachycardia or fibrillation occurring in 2.3%, and prolonged angina occurring in 6.7%. Long term follow-up of one year following angioplasty was assessed in 1,397 patients. At the end of one year, 72% of patients with a primary successful result did not require repeat angioplasty or bypass, and 12% required repeat dilatation. Therefore, 84% of patients with a primary successful result could be managed by angioplasty alone at the end of one year.

It must be emphatically stated that these results

represent "early" angioplasty prior to the widespread
availability of the newer guide wire--dilatation catheter
systems. Experienced operators using state of the art
equipment are approaching a 90% primary success rate,
although, the restenosis rates remain substantial (15-33%).

A particularly important application of transluminal
coronary angioplasty is in patients with evolving transmural
myocardial infarction[7-9]. The use of intracoronary
streptokinase in the early hours of evolving myocardial
infarction results in re-establishment of coronary flow in
approximately 75% of patients[10-12]; however, following intracoronary streptokinase therapy high grade residual stenoses
often remain and serve as sites for rethrombosis[13]. In an
attempt to achieve more long lasting results, investigators
have applied the technique of angioplasty to the residual
stenoses remaining in coronary arteries following successful
therapy with intracoronary streptokinase. For example, in a
series by Meyer et al, transluminal coronary angioplasty was
performed in 21 patients with acute myocardial infarction
treated by intracoronary streptokinase[8]. Thrombolysis
therapy was administered 3.6 $\pm$ 1.2 hours after symptom onset
and transluminal coronary angioplasty was performed 20-60
minutes after the end of the streptokinase treatment in 19
patients and 24 and 31 hours after treatment in 2 patients.
Angioplasty was successful in 17 of 21 patients. Twenty
patients survived hospitalization; an autopsy performed on
the patient who died in hospital revealed a patent infarct
related vessel. During the post hospital follow-up period
there were 2 reinfarctions and one asymptomatic reocclusion.
These results were compared to a "control" group of patients
with acute myocardial infarction who were treated with intracoronary streptokinase infusion alone. In the latter group
there were 4 in hospital reinfarctions and 3 patients died
furing the follow-up period. These investigators concluded
that transluminal coronary angioplasty could be performed
effectively and safely during evolving myocardial infarction;

that reocclusion rate is reduced and overall prognosis improved by the addition of angioplasty to intracoronary streptokinase therapy.

The technique of coronary angioplasty is still in a relatively early state of development; with increased operator experience and further improvements in technology, this exciting therapeutic modality will have an increasingly important role.

REFERENCES

1. Gruentzig AR, Senning A, Siegenthaler WE: Nonoperative
    dilatation of coronary artery stenosis percutaneous
    transluminal coronary angioplasty. N Engl J Med(301):61,
    1979.

2. Kent KM, Bentivoglio LG, Block PC, Cowley MJ, Dorros G,
    Gosslein AJ, Gruentzig A, Myler RK, Simpson J, Stertzer SH,
    Williams DO, Fisher L, Gillespie MJ, Detre K, Kelsey S,
    Mullin SM, Mock MB: Percutaneous transluminal coronary
    angioplasty: Report from the registry of the National
    Heart, Lung and Blood Institute. Am J Cardiol(49):2011,
    1982.

3. Cowley MJ, Vetrovec GW, Wolfgang TC: Efficacy of percu-
    taneous transluminal coronary angioplasty: Technique,
    patient selection, salutary results, limitations and
    complications. Am Heart J(101):272, 1981.

4. National Heart Lung and Blood Institute Registry Report,
    Nov. 1983.

5. Dervan JP, Baim DS, Cherniles J, Grossman W: Transluminal
    angioplasty of occluded coronary arteries: Use of a
    movable guide wire system. Circ(68):776-784, 1983.

6. Hartzler GO, Rutherford BD, McConahay DR: Simultaneous
    multiple lesion coronary angioplasty. A preferred
    therapy for patients with multiple vessel disease. Circ
    (66):(suppl II) II-5, 1982 (abstr.).

7. Goldberg S, Urban P, Greenspon AL: Combination therapy
    for evolving myocardial infarction: Intracoronary
    thrombolysis and percutaneous transluminal angioplasty.
    Am J Med(72):994, 1982.

8. Meyer J, Merx W, Schmitz H: Percutaneous transluminal
    coronary angioplasty immediately after intracoronary
    streptolysis of transmural myocardial infarction. Circ
    (66):905-913, 1982.

9. Hartzler GO, Rutherford BD, McConahay DR: Percutaneous
    transluminal coronary angioplasty with and without
    thrombolytic therapy for treatment of acute myocardial
    infarction. Am H J(106):965-973, 1983.

10. Rentrop P, Blanke H, Carsh KR, et al: Selective intra-
    coronary thrombolysis in acute myocardial infarction and
    unstable angina pectoris. Circ(63):304, 1981.

11. Mathey DG, Kuch KH, Tilsner V, et al: Nonsurgical
    coronary artery recanalization in acute transmural myo-
    cardial infarction. Circ(63):489, 1981.

12. Ganz W, Buchbinder N, Marcus H, et al: Intracoronary
     thrombolysis in evolving myocardial infarction. Am H
     J(101):4, 1981.

13. Urban P, Cowley M, Goldberg S, et al: Clinical course
     after myocardial reperfusion during myocardial infarction.
     Circ (III): Suppl III, 210, 1983 (abstr).

22

DEVICES TO LIMIT INFARCT SIZE: VENTRICULAR ASSIST DEVICES

JACK KOLFF, M.D.

INTRODUCTION

   The title of this presentation might well be changed into a
multiple choice question for a final examination in
bioengineering. The question would read: Ventricular assist
devices; limit infarct size, and improve myocardial function.
Mark (a) if both statements are true, (b) if both statements
are false; or, (c) if one statement is true and one is false.

   In order to address this question which in earlier days
might have been an essay question, I would like to review the
definitions of infarction and atrophy and present some basic
studies of muscle anatomy. You will then become aware through
the presentation of some clinical data that we have proceeded
with the use of these devices without knowing the full impact
and consequences of their use, which is not unlike the
transplanters proceeding with transplantation without having
solved the immunologic barrier, justifiably I might add.
Finally, I will outline a research study which might further
help identify the correct answer to the original question.

DEFINITIONS

A Myocardial Infarction is defined as death of a portion of cardiac muscle caused by metabolic alterations within a group of myocytes leading to destruction of all intracellular components and death of cells. A myocardial infarction is a consequence of an insufficient amount of energy supplies for the work load that the muscle is required to perform.

In myocardial atrophy, there is a decrease in the cross-sectional area and the volume of the cell. On closer examination a change is seen in the structure and composition of the intracellular elements including a disorientation and loss of contractile filaments and a loss of the "z" line substance. This results in altered functional capabilities.[1]

The difference between skeletal muscle and cardiac muscle is that atrophy of the skeletal muscle is seen with denervation of the muscle whereas cardiac mass is independent of neural factors. The transplanted heart, although denervated does not atrophy. Cooper and Tomanek suggest that there is strong evidence that cardiocyte mass and structure are "implicitly dependent upon stretch and/or tension".[2]

If an assist device can increase energy delivery, for example, by increasing diastolic aortic pressure and coronary flow, and/or decrease work load as, for example, by decreasing the afterload on the ventricle, it could theoretically limit the size of an ongoing infarction. The previous paper of the

Symposium has addressed this issue as it pertains to one device, the intra-aortic balloon pump. The dilemna is that when a ventricular assist device decreases the myocardial workload it induces atrophy and functional disability suggesting we shouldn't use a ventricular assist device when myocardial function is already impaired.

CASE PRESENTATION

Clinically, we have no choice. We have come to the end of the line. We are beyond the criteria for cardiogenic shock and intra-aortic balloon pumping.[3]

Case 1. A 63 year old white female with a history of hypertension, congestive heart failure, angina pectoris and chronic obstructive pulmonary disease and status post bilateral carotid endarectomy and aorto-femoral bypass was transferred to our hospital. Four days previous to transfer she had suffered an acute infero-posterior myocardial infarction complicated by pulmonary edema as well as acute renal failure attributed to hypotension. She had been started on peritoneal dialysis but developed peritonitis for which she was transferred for management. Pertinent physical findings: pulse of 84, blood pressure 150/90, respiratory rate 18, a jugular venous pressure of 7 cm. at 30°. The chest revealed diffuse rhonchi and scattered rales. She was in regular sinus rhythm with a variable intensity S1, a I/VI basal systolic ejection murmur and II/VI apical holo systolic murmur. The abdomen was diffusely tender with mild rebound and hypoactive bowel sounds. There was no rigidity or guarding.

Laboratory Studies: WBC 7.2, 61 segs, 14 bands, 9 lymphs, and 16 monocytes, Hgb 14.3, Hct 40.6, K 4.4, Cl 98, HCO_3 19, BUN 183 Creat 9.0, CPK 146, LDH 647, SGOT 63. The patient was anuric, the EKG showed sinus rhythm with alternating first and second degree AV block and infero-posterior myocardial infarction with diffused ST and T wave abnormalities. The chest X-ray revealed bi-basilar fluffy infiltrates. Arterial blood gases on 40% non rebreathing face masks were 76/94/32/18.4/7.38. The pulmonary capillary wedge pressure was 16 mm of mercury.

Hospital course - 1) Klebsiella peritonitis secondary to peritoneal dialysis resolved with antibiotic therapy; 2) Status post-myocardial infarction and acute renal failure - the patient's six weeks hospital course was complicated by repeated bouts of congestive heart failure and pulmonary edema. The thirtieth hospital day she suffered a cardiac arrest while being hemodialyzed attributed to hypotension. At this time, the murmur of mitral regurgitation was noted to have increased in intensity. The patient did poorly with medical management and underwent cardiac catheterization in search of a surgically correctable lesion. Severe mitral regurgitation was demonstrated and the patient underwent mitral valve replacement.

After mitral valve replacement the patient could not be weaned from the heart-lung machine because of right ventricular failure. Adequate left ventricular function was present. A right ventricular assist device was devised and the patient was eventually weaned from cardio-pulmonary bypass. Eight hours later right ventricular function recovered and the patient returned to the operating room for removal of the right ventricular assist device. Subsequently, she developed refractory hypoxemia, an arrhythmia and suffered a cardiac arrest. The hemodynamic course is illustrated in Figure 1. After right ventricular assist pumping for eight hours, hemodynamically she was stable enough to withdraw support.

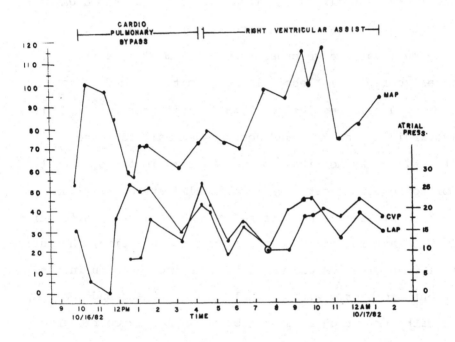

FIGURE 1. The hemodynamic course of a patient who underwent right heart assist. The patient demonstrated stability after eight hours at which time withdrawal was accomplished.

However, oxygenation became increasingly more difficult as shown in Figure 2 and eventually caused her demise. She might have been considered a candidate for extracorporeal membrane oxygenation if we had had an indication of a more favorable prognosis.

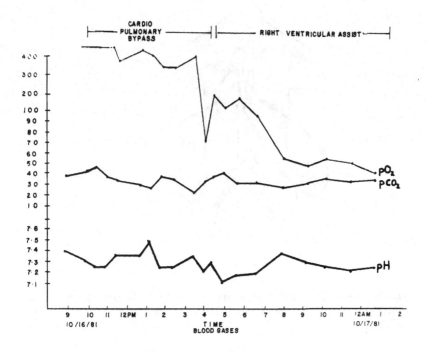

FIGURE 2. The results of blood gas analysis of a patient during right ventricular assist pumping. Although pCO_2 and pH were maintained within normal limits, oxygenation became increasingly difficult.

The circuitry that we have used for right as well as left bi-ventricular assist pumping consists of regular venous uptake tubing connected to high grade roller pump tubing and a return via standard arterial cannulas.[4] Figure 3 shows the combination of a right and left ventricular assist pump and can be equated to a heart-lung machine except for the fact that we use the patient's own lungs for gas exchange.

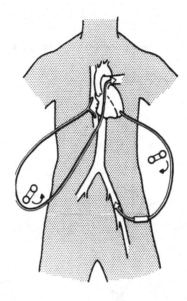

FIGURE 3. An illustration of the circuitry utilized during right and/or left ventricular assist pumping. Both circuits are used simultaneously for bi-ventricular assist.

Case 2. A 60 year old gentlemen who underwent triple coronary artery bypass grafting became hemodynamically unstable in the Intensive Care Unit and required the intra-aortic balloon. He remained in shock and was therefore taken back, placed on partial heart-lung bypass and then converted to biventricular assist support as illustrated in Figure 3. Figures 4 and 5 illustrate the hemodynamic course, in particular, it's noteworthy that the CVP and LAP could be maintained under 20 mm. of mercury. Biventricular assist allows complete control of blood flow through both the pulmonary and systemic circulations resulting in adequate perfusion of peripheral organs as indicated by the resumption of urine output. (Figure 5)

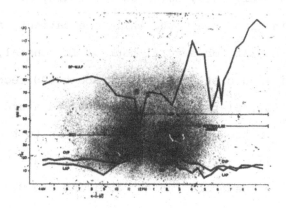

FIGURE 4.   The hemodynamic course of a patient who required bi-ventricular assist after becoming increasingly unstable following coronary artery surgery. Mean blood pressure improved significantly as well as maintaining the filling pressures within normal limits.

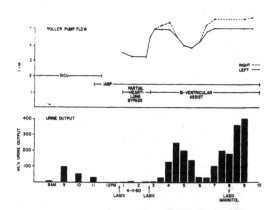

FIGURE 5.   This illustrates the renal failure associated with cardiogenic shock and hypotension in a patient prior to bi-ventricular assist.   As cardiac output and organ perfusion increased due to assist pumping, urine output improved greatly.

We, like other investigators, have had difficulty with some persistent bleeding from the wound while the patient is on uni- or biventricular assist for several hours. In general, we like to keep the "activated clotting time" at about 200 seconds, hematocrit above 25%, platelets above 20,000 and avoid excessive suctioning to try to keep plasma free hemoglobin to the lowest possible level. Clinically, during cardio-pulmonary bypass, we use only membrane oxygenators thereby avoiding the platelet and coagulation difficulties that might arise from long pump runs on bubble oxygenators. The hematologic data is shown in Figure 6. We terminated support when it became evident that the patient had sustained neurologic death during his episode of hypotension in The Surgical Intensive Care Unit.

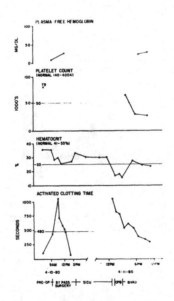

FIGURE 6. Hematologic studies of a patient who underwent coronary artery surgery followed by bi-ventricular assist. Although we have experienced difficulty in maintaining normal hematologic parameters, the use of a membrane oxygenator has allowed us to attempt much longer pump runs than could be accomplished with bubble oxygenators.

If biventricular assist is used relatively late after a
myocardial infarction and the patient has developed pulmonary
congestion it may take hours for the pulmonary damage to be
corrected, however, if biventricular assistance is used early and
there has been no chance for pulmonary edema to develop, then
the natural lungs can be used as an excellent oxygenator and
both pCO_2 and pO_2 can be normal. Figures 7 and 8 illustrate
data of a patient who required biventricular assist to maintain
hemodynamics immediately after coming off cardio-pulmonary
bypass. The inspiratory O_2 could be reduced to 45% keeping the
pO_2 above 100 mm Hg.

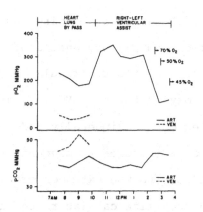

FIGURE 7. A patient who receives bi-ventricular assist as an early support
for post-myocardial infarction demonstrates an ability to oxygenate much
better. This is due to the fact that pulmonary edema did not have a chance
to develop and the natural lungs can perform with normal efficiency.

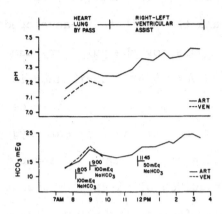

FIGURE 8. This illustrates the ability to maintain adequate perfusion due to good blood flow and oxygen supply on a patient supported with bi-ventricular assist in the early stages of a myocardial infarction.

Thus, adequate blood flow and normal hemodynamics can be maintained more easily with biventricular assist pumps than with only right or left ventricular assist pumping and in conjunction with non-diseased lungs can supply oxygenated blood to all organs.

The difference between using two ventricular assist pumps and extracorporeal membrane oxygenator or ECMO is that the venous uptake cannula is located more peripherally and in that the femoral bypass pump circuit includes an oxygenator. We have, on several occasions, been able to use extracorporeal membrane oxygenation in order to stabilize cardiac rhythm and blood pressure prior to the removal of massive pulmonary emboli. The hemodynamic course of one of these patients is illustrated in Figure 9.

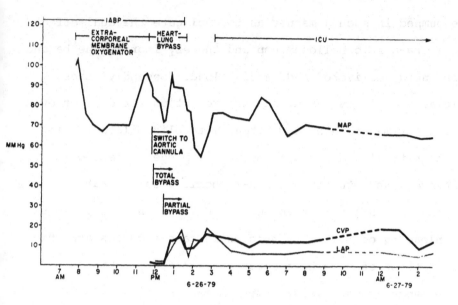

FIGURE 9. The hemodynamic course of a patient requiring ECMO. Patient stability and normal hemodynamic parameters are the results of utilizing ECMO in patients with CODD, and/or pulmonary embolus.

From our clinical experience we conclude that there is no doubt that we can support the entire circulation with ventricular assist pumps but because of the complexity and the considerable risks involved, this mode of treatment is not utilized until all other forms of treatment have been shown to be inadequate and the patient's death is imminent.

FUTURE STUDIES

The effect that these artificial ventricles have on the natural heart are several fold. First of all, the artificial ventricle can be pumped in such a manner as to duplicate the dual effect of the intra-aortic balloon pump and thereby improve the balance between energy delivered and cardiac load. Secondly, these artificial ventricles can maintain circulation for days or even weeks thereby maintaining the normal metabolic milleau during which the natural heart could recover from edema, metabolic disturbances, and other acute non-ischemic insults that may have caused the original threat to heart and life. However, because total unloading of papillary muscles in cats produces atrophic changes, these studies have important implications for semi-permanent ventricular assist pumps in man.

Our laboratory is initiating a human study that will hopefully shed some light on the rate atrophic changes occur in man. We have experimented with the implantation of a right ventricular assist pump located adjacent to the right atrial wall and thus are able to unload the right ventricle. The anatomical position-ing of such a ventricle in a human body is shown in Figure 10. Percutaneously obtained myocardial biopsies will be studied for changes in structure and composition of intracellular elements and these will be correlated with functional abnormalities obtained by computer monitoring of the hemodynamics as described by Stanley.[5] By unloading and later reloading the natural ventricle, atrophic changes could perhaps be minimized by circulatory support systems and hypertrophic changes could be induced during the recovery phase.

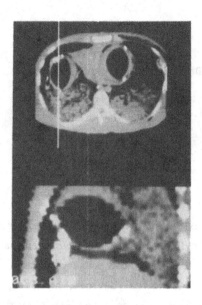

FIGURE 10. A computerized axial tomograph of a patient implanted with a right ventricular assist pump. The utilization of this tool helps determine exact anatomical positioning of such a ventricle in the human body.

REFERENCES

1. Cooper G, Tomanek RJ: Load Regulation of the Structure, Composition, and Function of Mammalian Myocardium, Circ Res (50):788-798, 1982.

2. Tomanek RJ, Cooper G: Morphological Changes in the Mechanically Unloaded Myocardial Cell. Anat Rec (200):271-280, 1981.

3. Corday E, Meerbaum S, Lang TW: Treatment of Cardiogenic Shock with Mechanical Circulatory Assist - Fact or Fiction? Am J Cardiol (30):575-578, 1972.

4. Watanabe K, Kabei N, McRea J, Peters J: Continuous Measurement of Myocardial Oxygen Consumption (MVO2) and Hemodynamic Response During Transapical Left Ventricular Bypass (TALVB). Trans Am Soc Artif Intern Organs (21):566-571, 1975.

5. Stanley T, Boam W: Use of the Computer to Monitor Long-Term Cardiac Assistance. J Thoracic & Cardiovasc Surg (57):519-526, 1969.

23

Internal Electrical Devices to Limit Infarct Size

Leonard N. Horowitz, M.D.

In other sections of this symposium pharmacologic and mechanical interventions which can limit infarct size have been discussed. Although there are no specific devices whose primary function would be to limit infarct size, internal electrical devices, however, can be used to optimize hemodynamic performance and reduce further necrosis which may be related to arrhythmias in the setting of acute myocardial infarction. By these means internal electrical devices can contribute to the limitation of infarct size. Such modalities include AV sequential pacing, pacing for termination of arrhythmias, and transvenous low energy countershock for termination of arrhythmias.

AV SEQUENTIAL PACING

The need for temporary cardiac pacing during acute myocardial infarction becomes necessary when transient or permanent complete heart block develops. Although ventricular demand pacing may be life-saving in this situation the consequences of the loss of atrial contribution to ventricular filling and altered ventricular contraction patterns in an already compromised left ventricle creates disadvantageous hemodynamic results. The advantages of AV sequential pacing which maintains AV synchrony and optimizes hemodynamic performance have been shown.[1,2] The advantages of AV sequential pacing is most marked in the setting of left ventricular dysfunction which is a prominent clinical feature in acute myocardial infarction. Although the clinical results of AV sequential pacing have not been specifically studied in patients with acute myocardial infarction, data obtained in patients with other cardiac disease states suggest that this pacing modality would be beneficial in optimizing hemodynamics and preventing further mechanical deterioration in post-infarction patients.

PACING FOR TERMINATION OF ARRHYTHMIAS

Pacing can also be used in the setting of acute myocardial infarction for prompt termination of both atrial and ventricular arrhythmias.[3,4] The advantages of arrhythmia termination utilizing pacing include the rapidity with which this modality can be applied, the avoidance of cardiodepresant effects of acute administration of antiarrhythmic and anesthetic agents, and the avoidance of transthoracic countershock. Atrial flutter and paroxysmal supraventricular tachycardia can be reliably terminated by bursts of rapid atrial pacing. Particularly when this is required on a repetitive basis the benefits are realized. The acute administration of antiarrhythmic drugs and transthoracic cardioversion particularly reduce left ventricular function and may contribute to the extension of infarct size. Prompt restoration of normal sinus rhythm will additionally reduce the potential for ischemically related left ventricular dysfunction and extension of myocardial necrosis due to the increased oxygen consumption produced by the rapid rate.

Sustained ventricular tachycardia, a not uncommon complication of acute myocardial infarction can frequently be terminated by overdrive pacing.[5,6] Again the advantages of rapid conversion without the need for transthoracic cardioversion provide the rational for its use. Occasionally a patient with acute myocardial infarction will develop an incessant ventricular tachycardia which can be managed by atrial overdrive pacing.[7,8] In this particular setting the restoration of AV synchrony increases cardiac output and blood pressure and can serve to limit the extension of the myocardial infarction. Ventricular pacing, however, is generally required for arrhythmia termination and can be accomplished with a temporary transvenous catheter.

TRANSVENOUS CARDIOVERSION

Ventricular pacing for termination of ventricular tachycardia in the setting of stable, chronic organic heart disease is frequently effective; however, in the setting of acute myocardial infarction, ventricular tachycardia is less often ammenable to this type of treatment. In post-infarction patients a more appealing treatment modality appears to be transvenous cardioversion.[9] In this technique a catheter is positioned in the right ventricular apex for use during the period of high arrhythmia frequency. Electrodes on this catheter are positioned in the right ventricle and right atrium and cardioversion can be achieved with reasonably low currents. Yee, et al [10] have reported the use of this technique in eight patients in a coronary care unit with recurrent ventricular tachycardia and ventricular fibrillation. Ninety-nine transvenous countershocks were delivered for 91 episodes of ventricular tachycardia. Sixty-five percent of the episodes of ventricular tachycardia were converted with less than 5 joules and 90% of episodes were converted with less than 10 joules of energy. This technique allows the cardioversion pulse to be delivered more rapidly than the transthoracic technique and appears to be associated with no more and possibly less myocardial depression and damage than with transthoracic cardioversion. This technique's principal advantages appear to lie in the rapidity with which the arrhythmia can be terminated and the lower energy delivered to the heart. With slow tachycardias the cardioversion can be achieved with less than 1 joule of energy. This technique, like rapid ventricular pacing for termination of ventricular tachycardia, can occasionally produce ventricular fibrillation. In such an eventuality either transvenous or transthoracic defibrillation is necessary.

Although no internal electrical device has been specifically developed which as a primary effect can reduce or limit infarct size, it is clear that the damaging effects that various brady and tachy-arrhythmias can be ameliorated with internal anti-tachycardia devices. Further investigation is necessary to establish the appropriate role and therapy of these devices and the development of newer devices with greater applicability. For the immediate future, internal electrical devices will, however, remain as an adjunctive means of treating myocardial infarction and limiting the extent of myocardial necrosis.

REFERENCES

1. Reiter MJ, Hindman MC: Hemodynamic effects of acute atrioventricular sequential pacing in patients with left ventricular dysfunction. Am J Cardiol. 49: 687, 1982
2. Leinbach RC, Chamberlain DA, Kastor JA, Hawthorne JW, Sanders CA: A comparison of the hemodynamic effects of ventricular and sequential AV pacing in patients with heart block. Am Heart J 78:502, 1969

3. Waldo AL, MacLean WAH, Karp RB, Kouchoukes NT, James TN: Entrainment and interruption of atrial flutter with atrial pacing. Studies in man following open heart surgery. Circulation 56:737, 1977

4. Spurrell RAJ, Sowton E: Pacing techniques in the management of supraventricular tachycardia. J. Electrocardiography. 8: 287, 1975

5. Josephson ME, Horowitz LN, Farshidi A, Kastor JA: Recurrent sustained ventricular tachycardia: I. Mechanisms. Circulation 57:431, 1978

6. Wellens HJJ, Schuilenberg RM, Durrer D: Electrical stimulation of the heart in patients with ventricular tachycardia. Circ. 46: 216, 1972

7. Horowitz LN, Josephson ME, Spielman SR, Greenspan AM, Harken AH: J. Cardiovas Med 5:715, 1980

8. DeSanctis RW, Kastor JA: Rapid intracardiac pacing for treatment of recurrent ventricular tachyarrhythmias in the absence of heart block. Am heart J 76:168, 1968

9. Zipes DP, Jackman WM, Heger JJ, Chilson DA, Browne KF, Naccarelli GV, Rahilly GI, Prystowsky EN: Clinical transvenous cardioversion of recurrent
life-threatening ventricular tachyarrhythmias: Low energy synchronized cardioversion of ventricular tachycardia and termination of ventricular fibrillation in patients using a catheter electrode. Amer Heart J. 103:789, 1982

10. Yee R, Zipes DP, Gulamhusein S, Kallok MJ, Klein GJ: Low energy countershock using an intravascular catheter in an acute cardiac care setting. Amer J Cardiol 50: 1124, 1982

24

DEVICES TO LIMIT INFARCT SIZE -- FDA EVALUATION

Glenn Rahmoeller

Introduction

The Federal Food, Drug, and Cosmetic Act (Act)
originated as the Food and Drug Act in 1906. The
Act has been amended many times since. One such
group of amendments, the Medical Device Amendments
of 1976 (Amendments), gave the FDA new
responsibilities and authorities for the regulation
of medical devices.

Among other provisions of the Amendments are
requirements that:

    (a)   a manufacturer notify (premarket
notification) FDA before it markets any
new device;

    (b)   FDA approve a premarket approval
application (PMA) for the marketing of
a new device that is significantly
different from devices that have been
marketed previously; and

    (c)   the local institutional review board
(IRB) and FDA approve an
investigational device exemption (IDE)
application for any clinical
investigation to determine the safety
or effectiveness of a new device.

In addition, FDA must also review and approve PMAs for
certain life-supporting and life-sustaining devices that
were marketed since before the Amendments, in order for
these devices to remain on the market. Detailed
descriptions of the procedures and the criteria for approval
of PMAs and IDEs have been published previously.[1-3]

The purpose of this presentation is to describe the
status of FDA approval of the following devices which are
intended to limit infarct size: percutaneous transluminal
coronary angioplasty (PTCA) catheters, intra-aortic balloon
(IAB) pumps and balloons, ventricular assist devices (VADs),
and non-implantable transvenous devices used for
cardioversion and antitachycardia pacing.

PTCA Catheters

Although transluminal angioplasty has been used for
dilating arteriosclerotic lesions in peripheral arteries
since 1964,[4] its use in coronary arteries did not begin
until 1977.[5,6] The FDA received its first PMA application
for a PTCA catheter in June 1979. That device was approved
for marketing in March 1980. Another PMA application for a
PTCA catheter was submitted to FDA in September 1981, and
subsequently approved in March 1982.

Both of these PMAs included in vitro data to show that
the materials used in the device are safe; the device is
sterile and non-pyrogenic; and that the physical properties
of the balloon catheter, such as its burst strength, are
appropriate for the intended use of the catheter. Animal
studies were performed to show that the catheter could be
advanced into the coronary circulation safely and

also to evaluate the effects of the PTCA procedure
histologically. Extensive clinical studies were performed
with each device to establish the patient selection criteria
and conditions under which the catheter can be used safely
and effectively.

The clinical study for the first PMA consisted of 285
procedures by 12 investigators, with follow-up for 6 months
or greater in 72 patients. In the study for the second PMA,
there were 193 attempted procedures in 172 patients by 16
investigators. There was 6 months or longer follow-up on 64
patients. In each case, the FDA approved the PMA on the
condition that (a) certain indications, contraindications,
and recommendations appear in the labeling; and (b) the
manufacturer provide for a continuing study to collect more
long-term results about the effectiveness of the procedure.

The following are examples of some of the labeling
requirements for PTCA catheters: (a) indications for single
vessel disease where the atherosclerotic lesion is
concentric, discrete, subtotal, non-calcific, and accessible
to a dilatation catheter; (b) a "relative" contraindication
for diffuse or calcified stenoses and for left main coronary
artery disease; (c) absolute contraindications for patients
who are not candidates for coronary artery bypass graft
surgery (since this may be necessary if there are
complications with the PTCA procedure); and (d)
recommendations for anticoagulant therapy during and
following the procedure, and recommendations that only
physicians with training in PTCA use these catheters.

I would like to discuss the importance of medical device labeling in general, and then specifically with regard to PTCA. I believe that labeling (the indications, contraindications, cautions, and warnings) is based on good scientific data. As such, it should be read and considered carefully by the clinician. In the case of the PMAs for PTCA catheters, I believe the guidance provided in the labeling was an important factor leading to FDA's approval. FDA believes that if this guidance is followed, the device is truly safe and effective. If, however, the indications, contraindications, and recommendations are not followed, it is expected that the clinical results would not show PTCA to be safe and effective.

Intra-Aortic Balloon Pumps and Balloons

Unlike PTCA catheters, intra-aortic balloon pumps and balloons (IAB devices or systems) were marketed before enactment of the Amendments (pre-Amendments devices). The Amendments require that manufacturers of certain life-supporting and life-sustaining pre-Amendments devices, such as IAB systems, submit PMAs to FDA at some time in the future. Each manufacturer will be required to submit data to show that his IAB device is safe and effective for its indicated uses in order to be allowed to continue to market his devices.

FDA may not require submission of these data for 4 or 5 years. PMAs for implantable pacemakers and artificial heart valves will probably be the highest priorities, and these may be requested within the next year. When FDA does request the PMAs for IAB systems, FDA will look for specific

indications for each device and the data to support those
indications. Therefore, if a manufacturer wants to indicate
the IAB device in the treatment of "unstable angina and
intractable angina which is refactory to pharmacologic
measures," and that "balloon pumping may significantly
reduce infarct size," then there must be data to support
those indications.

In the meantime, however, FDA has received premarket
notification submissions for 20 new IAB pumps and balloons
since 1976. FDA has determined that these new devices are
not significantly different from the pre-Amendments IAB
devices. The new devices were, therefore, permitted to be
marketed; but they will require PMAs at the same time that
FDA requires PMAs for the pre-Amendments IAB systems.

Ventricular Assist Devices

Ventricular assist devices (VADs) are different from
PTCA catheters and IAB systems in that VADs are still under
clinical investigation. Data are now being collected to
establish the conditions under which VADs are safe and
effective. For each study there must be a sponsor or
sponsor/investigator, investigator, and IRB. The sponsor
must submit an IDE to the IRB and FDA for approval before
initiating a clinical study. To approve a clinical
investigation, the IRB and FDA must determine that the
benefits to the patients and the knowledge to be gained from
the study outweigh any risks to the patients. Specific
details of the responsibilities of sponsors, investigators,
IRBs, and FDA are in FDA's regulations and have been
described previously.[1-3]

A very important aspect of IDEs for these, and other, devices is to design the clinical trial for a specific purpose. The size of the study (in terms of the number of procedures and investigators, duration of the study, patient selection criteria, and the scientific protocol) should be consistent with the purpose of the study. If the device is still in a research or developmental phase, then the study should be small and patient selection criteria designed to minimize the risks to the patients. If the study is intended to support a PMA for marketing approval, then the patient selection criteria should be consistent with the proposed indications for the device; and the size of the study should be large enough to provide statistically significant data to support the indications, but no larger than necessary to show that the device is safe and effective. Also, the investigators should be well qualified and the number of investigators limited. Generally, FDA is looking for data collected in recognized centers for comparison with data on alternative procedures or therapies from similar centers. FDA generally does not have the resources to monitor large studies which are intended to show "typical" results.

Non-Implantable Transvenous Devices for Cardioversion and Antitachycardia Pacing

These devices include (a) those that are marketed only for temporary use and (b) those that are being used only for clinical research for the purpose of developing implantable permanent devices. Transvenous devices that fall into the first category would be required to comply with PMA approval at some future date, such as is the case with IAB systems. Those devices that are under clinical investigation require IDE approval and are regulated as are VADs.

Summary

Significantly new devices, such as PTCA catheters, must be approved by FDA before they may be marketed. The manufacturers of these devices must submit data to show that the labeling accurately reflects the conditions under which the device can be used safely and effectively. Some life-supporting and life-sustaining devices, (such as IAB systems) that were marketed before premarket review by FDA was required, are required by law to be reviewed by FDA at some time in the future. At that time, the manufacturers of these devices must provide scientific data to support each indication in the labeling.

Clinical evaluations of new devices, such as VADs, must be approved by each local IRB and by FDA. The scientific protocol for a clinical study must be consistent with the purpose of the study.

References

1. Rahimtoola SH, Rahmoeller GA: The law on cardiovascular devices: the role of the Food and Drug Administration and physicians in its implementation. Circulation (62): 919-924, 1980.
2. Dahms DF: New device approval by the Food and Drug Administration. In Morganroth E, Moore EN (ed) Sudden cardiac death and congestive heart failure: diagnosis and treatment. Martinus Nijhoff Publishers, Boston, 1983, pp 227-235.

3. Cheitlin MD: Evaluation of devices for the prevention
    of sudden death: study design for safety and efficacy
    of the devices. In Morganroth E, Moore EN (ed) Sudden
    cardiac death and congestive heart failure: diagnosis
    and treatment. Martinus Nijhoff Publishers, Boston,
    1983, pp 221-226.
4. Dotter CT, Judkins MP: Transluminal treatment of
    arteriosclerotic obstruction: description of a new
    technique and a preliminary report of its application.
    Circulation (30): 654-670, 1964.
5. Gruntzig A: Transluminal dilatation of coronary -
    artery stenosis. Lancet: 263, 1978.
6. Gruntzig A, Senning A, Siegenthaler WE: Nonoperative
    dilatation of coronary-artery stenosis: percutaneous
    transluminal coronary angioplasty. N Engl J Med
    (301): 61-68, 1979.

25

DEVICES TO LIMIT INFARCT SIZE

Dr. Leonard Horowitz

Dr. Ruberio: Do you think that synchronization of profusion with diastole would have any further advantage?

Dr. Goldberg: We are now looking at that in great detail. We are trying to compare direct arteriovenous versus diastolic synchronized retroperfusion with a balloon device on the end of the retroprofusion catheter or just retroperfusing using a roller pump device with a variable flow rate. We are trying to demystify whether diastolic synchronized retroperfusion is important. I might also add, expanding on your question retroperfusion is an idea method of delivering pharmacologic agents to the site of action where myocardial ischemia and necrosis is ongoing. It may be that the reason for the lack of efficacy of many of the agents that have been used in the past during evolving infarction has been the lack of ability to deliver it to the site of action and this may be a method of influencing and enhancing the efficacy of these agents. That is something we are going to be looking at very closely as well.

Dr. Morganroth: One of the important problems that a manufacturer has is clear indication for a device. One indication for a device such as intraortic balloon pulsation or transluminalangioplasty is that it has a medical endpoint such as correcting unstable angina or preventing death. On the other hand the endpoint can be a change in a hemodynamic measurement. How should an investigatorchoose the end point? How do you do a controlled study in devices.

Dr. Goldberg: I think your question is well taken. I don't think we are going to have a controlled trial in angioplasty. First of all angioplasty has been compared to coronary bypass surgery, not to medical therapy and I think this is proper and correct and I don't think patients should be chosen on the basis of just having a lesion. I think your question is getting a little bit more complex than that. That is, how can we tell that a device is working and a device that has substantial risk to it. For example, an intraortic balloon pump or a coronary retroperfusion device and let's for example take your patient with unstable angina. Obviously one cannot perform a placebo controlled type of trial. I think a very simple way of looking at it would be to do a parallel experiment to what I showed you in one of the animals. That is device working-not working during an act of ischemic episode for example. You can ask the patient if he has pain. You can look at the electrocardiogram. We are using precordial mapping, 35 lead mapping system to estimate infarct size. We have correlations between epicardial precordial mapping and infarct size determination just on the basis of the electrocardiogram. So I think it depends on what end point you are measuring to design your trial. If you are looking at unstable angina, frequency of anginal attack, with device on and off, duration of anginal attack, alteration and hemodynamic and electrocardiographic parameters, I think all of these are methods of getting at it. Although it is a very imperfect way of looking at it for obvious reasons.

Dr. Morganroth: How does one view a heart valve (like the Starr Edwards valve) that has been on the market for many years? Now it appears that the device act is going to require within the next few months or so the need to put together the essential equivalent of an NDA to show efficacy and safety and have specific claims and a summary basis for such an approval. I am unclear as to how that type of data will be required to parallel what we have for drugs. If one searches the literature to look for studies that are well controlled, properly reported and with some statistical basis as we would do for a drug, that there may not be much data in that regard on devices. So is there going to be a different standard for devices, than for drugs in terms of the scientific firmness of the data?

Dr. Rahmoeller: Briefly, what we require now for a new heart valve is extensive _in vitro_ testing. Wear testing, fatigue testing to get some idea as to how the valves will wear. We have not been quite as sucessful at that with the new Bjork-Shiley valve where there have been quite a few strut fractures as we might have hoped, but that I think shows some of the problems that can exist with what appear to be minor manufacturing changes to the valve. So we ask for that and then we ask for clinical testing and generally on a new device we ask for extensive testing on about 100 valves, roughly 35 to 50 in the aortic and 35 to 50 in the mitral position with LDH data, haptoglobin catheterizations on something like 28 valves if we can get that many. Usually the smallest and largest in both the aortic and mitral positions and follow-up on the patients with blood data for a year. So that is what we get now. What we are going to have to do in the future is to propose in the federal register first that we are going to call for these pre-market proof applications for the old valves and then set a date as to when they are going to be required to be submitted in order for them to remain on the market. I think what we will be doing over the next year or so is working with the device manufacturers to explore some of the alternative ways in which one might supply data. Will data from the literature and data from effect reports that the manufacturer has be useful in lieu of some of the prospective studies that are now done and we will explore that way. One other comment I will make is that when the Congress passed the device law, there are several differences between the device law and the drug law which I think show a different philosophy in time and that is that effectiveness in the drug law is that a drug has to be safe and effective in order to go to market. In order to market a new device, one has to be reasonably assured that it is going to be safe and effective. Slight differences in the language. Efficacy in the drug law is based on well controlled clinical studies, and the device law is well controlled clinical studies or other valid scientific evidence. So when congress passed the medical device amendments, I think they were trying to weave into those a slight difference in philosophy to take into account some of the lags that they perceived.

Dr. Morganroth:: How do you view the data that document that devices used for the last decade are safe and effective? Is that something that would be relatively straight forward or is that going to be some problem from a scientific point of view?

Dr. Kolff: There are several difficulties. First of all, we must realize that whenever we come up with a new device, that it won't be the panacea, the perfect device, because we don't have the best possible material. Constantly materials are coming on the market which are better, stronger, or more resilient or less thrombogenic. It becomes very difficult sometimes to show in this particular biological environment, that a particular product will do better. You might do better on one aspect than on the other hand, you might lose a little. It is a trade off. You might lose a little strength, you might lose a little resilience. Let's say you take a clinically used device like a valve and you put it in a blood pump, one of these ventricular assist pumps and you find that these valves break. It is a little bit like the little boy closing the door. He enjoys closing the door, but you as the father think that the boy is closing the door too hard. He keeps slamming the door and eventually your suspicions are right, the door breaks so the carpenter puts in a heavier door. The frame breaks now when the kid slams the door. The carpenter is not the correct way to go about it. You have to spank the boy and say quit closing the door so hard. It is the dp/dt on that door that breaks it. Lastly, when you take a device and put it someplace else, a slightly different situation are all the scientific elements really looked at? That is something very difficult to come up with and I would hate to have somebody just direct somebody else by saying you got to use x,y,z valve because we think it is better. Is it really, probably not. Lastly to go from animals to humans or from species to species, we really know very little about what happens. For example, the old story is that if you would wait with the devlopment of valves and prove it in animals first, gee, you might never get a valve into a human subject. If you take a valve and you put it into somebody, then perhaps it will work.

Dr. Morganroth: Dr. Horowitz, what problems do you forsee in going back to look at the VVI pacemakers to document efficacy and safety for these marketed devices?

Dr. Horowitz: My assumption is that all of DDD pacemaker were reviewed under the current regulations so it is only a matter of reviewing the VVI pacemakers. This is reasonably simple because you have to show that it paces the heart and that it senses. I think that is easily done scientifically. To prove that it works, I would suspect that the FDA is not going to require companies that it is better to be paced than unpaced if you have a symptomatic bradyarrhythmia. I think that aspect is fairly straight forward.

Dr. Rahmoeller: I would like to make one point as a follow-up to the
Shiley valve because I think it is important. That valve went through
pre-market approval. It has been modified by manufacturing process or
quality-control process three times. From the first time to the secondtime,
it was a quality control process, a non-destructive type of test was applied
hopefully to eliminate the problems with downstream strut fracture. It
turns out that based on the actuarial data we have now and just received
about a week or two ago, that the two year actuarial rate for strut fracture
of the Shiley valve, the first model that was approved under the PMA is less
than 1/10th of 1%. The downstream strut fracture actuarial at 2 years for
the second model which has already gone recall is .74% and so it appears to
be a good change is not necessarily good change and I think what you have to
do is just go back to some of these valves and look and see what is the
thromboembolic complication rate, what is the explant rate, at least within
certain patient groups.

Dr. Temple: I think you are setting up a little red herring to wonder
about placebo controlled trials of whether a valve is there. That is just
not necessary. It is not a necessary element of study design to see whether
it allows blood to go forward and keeps it from going back. I mean you
don't need a placebo for that. You have more than an adequate historical
control data to say that without the artifact there is no pace, or in many
cases, some of the questions start to get interesting. Whether they are
prerequisites for approval or not I don't know, but one does want to know I
think whether a transvenous angioplasty or something like that, how does
that compare with doing nothing, doing a bypass graft procedure and things
like that? Those are sort of big questions and one could have them to
debate I think about whether that should be done before marketing or after
marketing.

Dr. Morganroth: The analogy to that concept it seems to me is the PVC
question in sudden death. That is if the efficacy is defined as simple
reduction in PVC's by a new antiarrhythmic drug, that would be to me like
saying that a PTCA or angioplasty has to show only a hemodynamic change.

Dr. Temple:I think it depends on an intuitive judgement that there could be
something wrong with the procedure so that obviously people looked at

suppression of VPB's and they said I am not sure what the effect of this on life is, but it doesn't look like it can be bad. That may not be true. Some further effect of the drug may indeed be bad and I think the same kind of reasoning goes with all of these other procedures. If you can speculate on a lot of ways that could turn out to be worse than doing nothing, you probably do have to ask the hard questions. If you can't think of any ways, I guess the inclination is to let them go.

Dr. Rahmoeller: You have to ask what the question is first and I think the manufacturers at first brought the PTCA to the FDA were really asking the wrong questions. It wasn't only in talking to some of the investigators that I think we made a case for it. That is the morbidity and mortality of PTCA is no better than it is with coronary artery bypass surgery. The real benefit of it is that if you can postpone the initial bypass operation then you postponed a second bypass operation and you are dealing with in this case younger patients, 39,40,45 age group. What the panel approved was if all you could do was buy 6 months to a year of postponing that first bypass operation that it is useful. We don't have to determine whether it is cost effective or not, but it was useful. The other thing was when you talk about safety and effectiveness, I think it is good to break it down into short term effectiveness, long term safety, long term effectiveness and look at it that way. It is a little more complicated if you jumble it up.

Dr. Temple: That is a good example. There is substantial debate about when various procedures are effective in what subgroups they are effective, in who they should be used and these are not by any means settled issues. People with one lesion have generally good cardiac dynamics and it isn't clear if they deserve any procedure or at least some people would say they don't. People who do them I guess think that is settled. Those are all questions one could ask in the course of deciding of whether to approve a device and how to label it.

Rahmoller::   It may be a lot different in that without devices we have no control over e.g. bypass operations at all. Coronary artery bypass surgery is at the discretion of the physicians.

Dr. Temple: The surgeons are grateful for that I understand.

Dr. Kolff: We love you for it because you decided that you go ahead and do a transluminal dilatation of the coronary occlusion and now all of a sudden we are seeing patients with single vessel disease that we wouldn't have operated on before. So the indications are changing. In someone with single vessel disease, coronary bypass grafting 0.1% operative mortality and you would be hard pressed to find a 0.1% operative mortality rate with PTCA.

Dr. Moore: I seem to remember at one of these meetings several years ago that when we were talking about antiarrhythmic drugs and beta blockers that it was brought up that in order to approve a new antiarrhythmic agent or a new beta blocker, that that drug should have some novel, or new advantage over the currently available antiarrhythmics and beta blockers. For example, pacemakers are very generic in many ways. Is there any aspect like that to the device regulation?

Dr. Rahmoeller: No there is not. We are required by law to use an advisory committee of physicians to review the applications that come and the direction is are you reasonably sure that the device is safe and effective. It is not a matter of comparing it and saying it is better, it is whether given those indications and contraindications in the labeling whether the advisory committee and the FDA believe that it is appropriate to market the device and as Dr. Kolff said, you are going to have a lot of trade-offs. Some devices are going to have some advantages and then some disadvantages and I think the big value that FDA has in this process is not whether it approves the device or doesn't approve the device, it is more often whether or not the limitations of the device are discerned and defined and then appropriately put in the labeling so that the physician that picks it up can understand what the limitations are. I think that is probably the most productive thing that we do.

Dr. Morganroth: Dr. Templet when you have to decide on, for example a 12th new beta blocker what is the policy of the cardio-renal division on handling such issues? Do you sort of put it at the bottom of the pile or do you just handle it without concerning yourself with the issue of drug redundancy?

Dr. Temple: There are two questions in there. One is, are we supposed to approve it even though we don't think it offers any advantage and the legislative history is very clear that we are. It could even be worse in some respects. We are supposed to approve it with accurate labeling. Do we rush it through, put it to the top of the pile? No, of course not, there are people probably still in the room who could tell you that, but the standard for approval does not involve a relative effectiveness requirement, so that is very clear from the legislative history so you don't have to be better. It turns out once there are a number of products available on the market place that enthusiasm for spending the many millions of dollars it takes to bring a drug to market is not very great for a product that doesn't have at least some potential advantage so you tend not to see them after a while. I think that is going one now for beta blockers with occasional exceptions.

SUMMARY OF SYMPOSIUM ON NEW DRUGS AND DEVICES

E. Neil Moore

This has been a very exciting and informative meeting. Dr. Reimer told us that if we don't do something by 3 hours after an MI that the cardiac cells are going to be irreversibly damaged. We also heard about a lot of very sophisticated ways to define infarct size such as electrocardiographic, echocardiographic, enzymatic, positron tomography and radionuclides. All of these methods under optimal circumstances can predict in a reasonably quantitative way, how much of the myocardium is actually infarcted. But conditions have to be very optimal, otherwise all of the infarct sizing techniques break down particularly when you have multiple infarctions, hypertrophy or other cardiac problems. It was very interesting to hear whether lidocaine, streptokinase, the vasodilators, and the calcium blockers can improve cardiac performance during and after an MI. I think that none of these compounds have been as good as we would like them to be. Dr. Campbell pointed out when you consider all the different evaluations that have been done on a given drug that you often find that the clinical trial aren't as nice and clean as you might like. In some ways that is not bad because if the pharmaceutical companies had been so fortunate as to find the magic bullets to get rid of all cardiac problems then many of us would be out of a job. It has been said that digitalis has probably created more jobs than lives it has saved. I think there is some truth to that. The comment that some drugs are given as much because they have few side effects as for their direct cardiac effects also has some truth.

We all await new guidelines in the evaluation of cardiac devices and I am sure that the years ahead will prove most interesting and challenging.

SYMPOSIUM ON NEW DRUGS AND DEVICES

October 6 & 7, 1983

Participant List

Cynthia B. Altman, M.D.
Director, Project Management and Strategic Planning
SmithKline Beckman Corporation

Keiko Aogaichi, M.D.
Senior Research Physician
Hoffmann-LaRoche, Inc.

Carla Ballard
Cardiovascular Product Manager
Smith Kline & French Laboratories

Mirza M. A. Beg, M.D.
Group Director of Planning & Operations
Smith Kline & French Laboratories

Edward Berman, M.D.
Bristol-Myers Company

Robert S. Brown
Director of New Studies
Cardio Data Systems

Larry R. Bush
Senior Research Pharmacologist
Merck Institute for Therapeutic Research

Catherine Cabot, M.D.
Ciba-Geigy Corporation

Ronald W. F. Campbell, M.D.
Senior Lecturer and Consultant Cardiologist
Freeman Hospital, England

Robert J. Capone, M.D.
Associate Professor of Medicine
Brown University

Rita A. Carey, Ph.D.
SmithKline Beckman Corporation

K. Cartwright, M.D.
Director, Clinical Research (USA)
Lederle Laboratories

Jay N. Cohn, M.D.
Professor of Medicine
University of Minnesota

David L. Copen, M.D.
Associate Clinical Professor of Medicine
Yale University

Willie Mae Coram, M.D.
Ciba-Geigy Corporation

James C. Costin, M.D.
Associate Director, Medical Affairs
ICI Americas, Inc.

Glenn G. Cousins
Research Division Manager
Cardio Data Systems

Michael Davidov, M.D.
Falls Church, Virginia

Philip Dern, M.D.
Cardio-Renal Division
Food and Drug Administration

Joseph R. DiPalma, M.D.
Professor of Pharmacology and Medicine
Hahnemann University

Stewart J. Ehrreich, Ph.D.
Deputy Director
Food and Drug Administration

Charles A. Ellis, Jr., M.D.
Andover, Massachusetts

J. L. Fischetti, M.D.
ICI Americas, Inc.

Gerald Eisen
Janssen Pharmaceutica

LaDean English
Methodist Hospital

Maria Geczy, M.D.
Syntex Laboratories

Kenneth M. Given, M.D.
Executive Director, Regulatory Affairs-Domestic
Merck Sharp & Dohme Research Laboratories

Herman Gold, M.D.
Associate Professor of Medicine
Harvard Medical School

Sidney Goldstein, M.D.
Professor of Medicine
University of Michigan

Leonard M. Gonasun, Ph.D.
Associate Director, Medical Research
Sandoz, Inc.

Ronald Goode, Ph.D.
Pfizer Pharmaceuticals

Richard Gorlin, M.D.
Chairman, Department of Medicine
The Mount Sinai Medical Center

William F. Graney, M.D.
Assistant Clinical Research Director
E. R. Squibb and Sons, Inc.

Allan M. Greenspan, M.D.
Associate Professor of Medicine
Hahnemann University

Juan R. Guerrero, M.D.
Medical Research Director
Knoll Pharmaceutical Company

Donald C. Harrison, M.D.
William G. Irwin Professor of Cardiology
Stanford University School of Medicine

Arthur H. Hayes, Jr., M.D.
Former Commissioner
Food and Drug Administration

Richard H. Helfant, M.D.
Professor of Clinical Medicine
University of Pennsylvania

Marc Henis, M.D.
Executive Director, Cardiovascular Clinical Research
Ciba-Geigy Corporation

John Hermanovich, M.D.
Assistant Professor of Medicine
Hershey Medical Center

Leonard N. Horowitz, M.D.
Associate Professor of Medicine
Hahnemann University

Alexis Lungendorf
Merck, Sharp & Dohme Research Laboratories

Richard F. MacIntosh
Product Manager
Astra Pharmaceutical Products, Inc.

Sara Armstrong Mahler, M.D.
Associate Medical Director
E. I. duPont deNemours & Company

Bernard F. McDonagh, Ph.D.
Market Development Manager
Riker Laboratories, Inc.

Charles F. McNally, M.D.
Director, Cardiovascular/Renal Group
Smith Kline & French Laboratories

Wolf D. Michaelis, M.D.
Hoechst-Roussel Pharmaceuticals, Inc.

Howard Miller, M.D.
Medical Director
Sandoz, Inc.

E. Neil Moore, D.V.M., Ph.D.
Professor of Physiology in Medicine
University of Pennsylvania

Joel Morganroth, M.D.
Professor of Medicine and Pharmacology
Hahnemann University

Manfred Mosk, Ph.D.
President, Medco Research
California

Cathleen B. Mullen, B.S.N.
Clinical Research Associate
Philadelphia Association for Clinical Trials

Gerald V. Naccarelli, M.D.
Assistant Professor of Medicine
University of Texas Medical School at Houston

Charlotte Anne Panis
Clinical Research Scientist
Sandoz, Inc.

Alfred F. Parisi, M.D.
Associate Professor of Medicine
Harvard Medical School

Indravadan I. Patel, M.D.
Research Physician
Hoffmann-LaRoche, Inc.

William S. Pickens, M.D.
Pensacola, Florida

Craig M. Pratt, M.D.
Assistant Professor of Medicine
Baylor College of Medicine

Glenn A. Rahmoeller
Director, Division of Cardiovascular Devices
Food and Drug Administration

Irwin M. Reich, M.D., Ph.D.
Assistant Medical Director
Sandoz, Inc.

Keith A. Reimer, M.D., Ph.D.
Associate Professor of Pathology
Duke University Medical School

K. Peter Rentrop, M.D.
Associate Professor of Medicine
Mt. Sinai Medical Center

R. E. Robinson, M.D.
Associate Global Medical Director
Merrell Dow Pharmaceuticals, Inc.

Rose M. Rogan, M.D.
Associate Medical Director
Organon, Inc.

Alberto Rosenberg, M.D.
Vice President, Clinical Research
Stuart Pharmaceuticals, Inc.

Elliott Rosenberg, M.D.
Assistant Professor of Medicine
Hospital of the University of Pennsylvania

John J. Schrogie, M.D.
Executive Director
Philadelphia Association for Clinical Trials

Ellen N. Sappington, R.N., M.S.
Merck Sharp & Dohme Research Laboratories

Peter Sleight, M.D.
Field-Marshall Alexander Professor of Cardiovascular Medicine
University of Oxford

Burton E. Sobel, M.D.
Professor of Medicine
Washington University School of Medicine

John C. Somberg, M.D.
Assistant Professor of Medicine
Albert Einstein College of Medicine

Scott R. Spielman, M.D.
Associate Professor of Medicine
Hahnemann University

Howard R. Steinberg, M.D.
Pfizer Pharmaceuticals

Anna Sweeney, M.D.
Merck, Sharp & Dohme Research Laboratories

Donald D. Suko
Ciba-Geigy Corporation

Michael J. Tansey, M.D.
Hoechst Aktiengesellschaft
Germany

John D. Teller
The Upjohn Company

Robert Temple, M.D.
Acting Director, New Drug Evaluation
Food and Drug Administration

Zoltan Turi, M.D.
Assistant Professor of Medicine
Harvard Medical School

Ilhan H. Tuzel, M.D.
Associate Director of Medical Research
Hoffmann-LaRoche, Inc.

Thomas L. Wenger, M.D.
Senior Clinical Research Scientist
Burroughs Wellcome Co.

James Willerson, M.D.
Professor of Medicine
University of Texas Health Science Center

Raymond L. Woosley, M.D., Ph.D.
Associate Professor of Medicine and Pharmacology
Vanderbilt University Medical Center

Phillip M. Young, Pharm.D.
Senior Clinical Research Associate
Marion Laboratories, Inc.

Gerald R. Zins, Ph.D.
Manager, Cardiovascular Diseases Research
The Upjohn Company